UNDERSTAN

Wendy Cooper

Understanding Osteoporosis

Every woman's guide to preventing
brittle bones

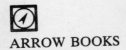

ARROW BOOKS

Arrow Books Limited
20 Vauxhall Bridge Road, London SW1V 2SA

An imprint of Random Century Group

London Melbourne Sydney Auckland Johannesburg
and agencies throughout the world

First published in 1990
Reprinted 1991

Printed and bound in Great Britain by
Courier International Ltd, Tiptree, Essex

ISBN 0 09 970620 2

Contents

Foreword

by Dr Allan Dixon OBE MD FRCP
Chairman of the National Osteoporosis Society

It must be deeply satisfying for Wendy Cooper to see her vision coming true – her vision of a country where women no longer have to suffer the debilitating symptoms and the premature ageing that is known as the menopause.

It is to her, if to anyone in this country, that the credit should be given for making the public and the medical profession first aware that the menopause and its consequences were preventable misfortunes, biologically out of tune with the vastly increased expectation of life that modern medicine and public health measures have brought for women.

In primitive societies, it may have made some kind of sense for women to die when they could no longer produce children. Today they may live half of their lives after their ovaries fail, and with the degenerative effects of oestrogen deficiency at work.

Wendy's pioneering book, *No Change*, drew attention to this and amongst the converted were a few doctors and surgeons dealing with women's problems who were prepared to take up the fight in the face of public ignorance and medical resistance.

Today the battle has been won. HRT has arrived. Wendy's title *No Change* proved paradoxical because it led to a great change – in attitudes toward the menopause and the treatment offered – and to the opportunity for women to enjoy increased quality of life as well as increased duration.

With this second book, the perfect follow up to *No Change*, Wendy tackles the most serious of all the effects of the oestrogen withdrawal, which nature has so unkindly arranged for women – the accelerated bone loss that occurs after the menopause and which leads to osteoporosis.

The problem is enormous. Osteoporosis related fractures now cost the country £800 million every year. The lion's share of this cost is attributable to fracture of the neck of the femur, or 'hip fracture', a disaster which in elderly women carries a fifteen per cent mortality rate. Premature osteoporosis in the 'not-so-old', the fifties, sixties and seventies, often strikes the spinal bones, leading to deformity, disability and pain. Wendy Cooper's message is: THIS IS ALL PREVENTABLE.

But, of course, it is not being adequately prevented. In a recent survey, published in the *British Medical Journal* (*BMJ*), of women who had had both ovaries removed for medical reasons, putting them at extremely high risk of developing osteoporosis, seventy per cent had never been treated with Hormone Replacement Therapy (HRT). Yet this is the *only* recognized method of stopping osteoporosis in its tracks. Even for the minority who were treated, oestrogen was prescribed on average for only twenty-one months – better than nothing, but not nearly long enough.

Many doctors now feel that failure to give women HRT following a surgical menopause is unethical. Some have even described it as criminally negligent. If so, four out of five of these women were criminally neglected.

So although HRT has long since been accepted by the informed doctor and even recommended by the Royal College of Physicians as the one effective means of stemming the rising tide of osteoporotic hip fractures in women, clearly there is still a need to raise the awareness of some doctors.

For this reason, in 1986 I helped set up the National Osteoporosis Society (NOS). Improvement of health education at all levels is badly needed and forms a big part of our work. NOS has to ensure that everyone – especially doctors – recognizes that osteoporosis is a preventable disease, not just another inevitable effect of getting older.

Family doctors have a key role to play in the battle against osteoporosis. They are in the best position to advise, prescribe and supervise HRT and, above all, explain its benefits and preventative role against brittle bones. And it is the GP who can most often identify those who are particularly at risk, for whom prophylactic treatment is going to be essential if they are to avoid the misery of osteoporotic fractures and deformity in later life.

Prevention is the message of this book and prevention implies prediction. Without the foreknowledge of what is going to happen to them if nothing is done, women are not going to demand that something *is* done. It was pressure from determined and motivated women who persuaded British medicine that it was time to consider greater availability of HRT. It will be pressure from women again that will achieve its wider usage now to combat brittle bones.

Introduction – alerting all women

Women are the main victims of osteoporosis – the medical term for 'porous bones'. Over the age of fifty, a quarter of us go on to develop this condition, with our bones becoming so thin and brittle that they fracture after only a light fall. If we live beyond seventy (and most women do in the developed world), *half* of us end up with actual osteoporotic fractures.

Unfortunately, 'end up' can in many cases be the all-too-appropriate term where the most dangerous of these fractures are concerned. Thinning bone at the narrow neck of the femur (thigh bone) now leads to some 52,000 older women sustaining fractured hips every year in Britain alone. And fifteen per cent of them (almost 8000) will die within six months from resultant complications.

Even for those who survive, the quality of life is poor, too often shadowed by pain, haunted by the increased threat of further fractures and limited by dependence on others. Half of the women who suffer hip fractures never again manage to lead independent lives.

Obviously all fractures are painful but where osteoporosis attacks the spine, there can be intense bouts of backache for years before the condition is diagnosed. By then it's often too late to prevent crushed and crumbling vertebrae, leading to loss of height and permanent ugly deformities, that are difficult to cope with physically and emotionally.

It's impossible to estimate the cost of osteoporosis to women in terms of this sort of human suffering, but to the NHS in terms of money and resources the cost is clear. It runs at over £500 million every year and it is rising! Visit any hospital and you'll find large numbers of beds in female surgical wards filled with hip-fracture patients, which means waiting lists for other less-urgent orthopaedic surgery, such as hip replacements, grow ever longer.

Significantly, the incidence of osteoporosis in *both* sexes is rising at a higher rate than can be accounted for merely by our increasingly ageing population, so that other aspects of modern life are clearly implicated. Some of these aspects are identified and remedies are suggested later in the book.

In January 1989, the Royal College of Physicians drew attention to this worsening situation in a special report on what they termed 'the osteoporosis epidemic'. It specially highlighted hip fractures in women and the fact that the sheer numbers involved were now so overwhelming that available hospital resources could often only provide very second-class treatment. The report urged more appropriate action be taken to protect women against brittle bones – in particular advocating the wider use of Hormone Replacement Therapy (HRT).

And that is where the good news comes in. In women, hormone replacement after the menopause can halt osteoporosis in its tracks. Used in good time, which is as soon as possible after the ovaries fail (natural menopause) or are removed (surgical menopause), HRT prevents the accelerated bone loss which otherwise occurs once the protection given to bone by female hormones is lost. *Restoring the hormones restores protection*.

Once established, osteoporosis cannot be cured or bone already lost be put back, except in certain circumstances and to a certain degree. So the message of this book is *prevention* and, for women, that essentially means HRT. Today, medical opinion worldwide accepts Hormone Replacement Therapy as the only proven effective method of preventing brittle bones in women and reducing the very real risk of painful and sometimes life-threatening fractures. In **Statements and Quotes from Doctors**, page 143, you will find this acceptance repeated again and again by leading doctors in this country.

HRT has already had a great deal of coverage in the media, not all of it full enough to be entirely accurate, and as a result certain myths and misconceptions have arisen. Hopefully you will find these dispelled in this book. Here you will find the facts about HRT and, for those who want them, the medical references to support them.

Chapter Five, page 67, explains in detail exactly what HRT is, how it works, what it does to relieve the more obvious physical and psychological menopause symptoms and, most important, how it counters the 'silent' insidious and serious symptoms that we are most concerned with here – dangerous post-menopausal bone loss.

In the details of British research carried out in our NHS menopause clinics, which has made HRT today so much safer and simpler to prescribe and to use, you will, I hope, find considerable reassurance. This chapter also describes the various different ways in which HRT can now be taken, and compares their relative advantages and disadvantages.

Of course, it would be foolish to overlook the fact that there's more to protecting bone than just replacing missing hormones, although that remains the vital protective factor for women. But for both sexes there are other positive and negative influences at work in our modern lifestyles that affect bone loss. These are also dealt with because we need to know about them and *use* that knowledge if we're each to *achieve* the maximum potential adult bone mass determined by our genes, and *maintain* it as far as possible against the normal effects of ageing – and in women against the onslaught of the menopause.

Diet comes high on the list of considerations, in particular, the need for adequate calcium intake throughout life but, most importantly, in our early years when bone mass is forming.

Chapter Six looks at the role of weight-bearing exercise, as vital to strong bones as it is to strong muscles and as simple to achieve as simply taking regular walks. This obvious form of exercise, undertaken by our ancestors right to the turn of this century, to the great benefit of their bones, has been neglected in our own age when time is money and swifter mechanized transport is readily available.

Other important adverse factors discussed include smoking, alcohol and a variety of drugs that act as 'bone robbers' both among those prescribed by doctors and those available over the counter. And for those already having to live with osteoporosis, the last two chapters offer practical guidance and real promise for the future. The latest treatments such as calcitonin and etidronate are described and their notes discussed.

There is an old adage about 'knowing your enemy'. And osteoporosis is your enemy and mine. So the more we know about it and the better we understand the influences at work, including the crucial role of the menopause in producing increased bone loss, and of Hormone Replacement Therapy in preventing it, the sooner this particular enemy will be defeated. Armoured with modern diagnostic techniques and preventative strategies, we now have the means the ensure that the familiar stereotype of 'the little old lady' recedes into the past.

Chapter 1

The female factors

While one woman in four is destined to develop osteo-porosis, a similar fate awaits only one man in forty and usually much later in life.

Quite obviously some special female factors are at work to account for such a difference between the sexes, and developments in modern medical knowledge mean there's no great mystery about them.

In the first place, men possess a heavier skeletal structure, with bones less vulnerable to thinning and the risk of fracture. But the most crucial difference lies in the fact that men have been allowed to evolve without running into a physical menopause in midlife, which brings about the loss of sex hormones and the vital protection these are now known to give to bone.

Testosterone in men and the ovarian hormone, oestrogen, in women, have been found to play similar essential roles in protecting bone. The sex hormones appear vital in preserving the critical balance between two opposing processes that go on throughout our lives – the formation of new bone and the resorption of old bone.

The complex interaction of hormones that controls this constant turnover of bone is discussed fully in Chapter Two. But for the moment, it's obvious that the female menopause and the resultant loss of protective sex hormones is bad news for bones.

The whole process is relentless. As ovaries fail, there is first a fall in progesterone and then in oestrogen, followed by a dramatic rise in bone loss. This loss is at its greatest during the first five to ten years immediately following the menopause. Afterwards there is some levelling off again, but by then considerable damage may have been done.

The degree of damage depends very much on how fast this accelerated bone loss occurs. This *rate* of loss varies from woman to woman, averaging some two to three per cent each year. It can, however, be as high as five per cent in what are termed 'fast bone losers'. The result is that ten to fifteen years into the menopause, most women will have lost thirty per cent of their bone mass, and the unfortunate fast bone losers may have lost as much as fifty per cent.

One of the most sinister aspects of this particular menopause symptom is our complete unawareness of what is happening. There is no warning; the process is 'silent', the progress insidious, and the first indication of trouble may be a deformity or a fracture.

Wrists, hips and vertebrae are the most vulnerable areas. Loss of height with bent, painful backs and the so-called dowager's hump can be familiar reminders of osteoporosis at work on the spine. Hip fractures not only disable, but cause more deaths in older women than cancers of the ovary, cervix and womb combined.[1]

But *why* has nature penalized women in this way? Why should men be allowed to retain adequate levels of sex hormones and enjoy the wellbeing and protection they confer while women are denied similar benefits?

Such basic sex discrimination seems grossly unfair, but nature takes the broader view. Anything built into the human blueprint by evolutionary forces has to be of benefit to the species as a whole and in some way favour its survival. So what were the advantages to the human race of setting a limit to female fertility? Why should orders for the shut-down of the ovaries in midlife (or earlier) become part of the genetic code for every human female?

Modern medicine has pinpointed the answer. Female babies are born complete with their lifetime supply of eggs and these eggs are known to deteriorate with age. This is clearly illustrated in the increased incidence of chromosome defects such as Down's syndrome (mongolism) in babies born to older mothers.

So, setting a limit to female fertility at least helped to limit the ever-increasing chance of substandard eggs being fertilized. It also helped to prevent children being born to mothers who might not live long enough to rear them (in the past the average life expectancy was short for women who were repeatedly exposed to the dangers of pregnancy, and the human child is dependent for many years).

With men, the situation was quite different. The male contribution to new life, the sperm, is freshly manufactured throughout life, and therefore no parallel advantage was to be gained by limiting male fertility. Accordingly, men were allowed to carry on producing sex hormones and fathering children (at least in theory) to the end of their lives.

Continued production of sex hormones brought men many advantages beyond prolonged fertility. For example, they age quite differently and less drastically than women. Men don't suddenly lose muscle tone and subcutaneous fat (fat immediately below the skin) from legs and arms, which causes the flabbiness common to so many women. Male skin doesn't undergo a drying and wrinkling process as early as ours, despite the potions and lotions we use to try and counteract the process. But most importantly, men don't suffer a sudden dramatic rise in bone loss so early in life that they become victims of brittle bones, fractures, bent backs and loss of height. No one talks of 'little old men' but people do speak rather pityingly of 'little old ladies'.

Today, at least, women have a chance to even things up. For the first time in history, the opportunities exist (if we want to use them) to overcome natural forms of sex discrimination just as they exist at last to overcome the manmade kind.

The two, needless to say, are related. When Freud declared that 'biology is destiny' he was absolutely right. It was basic female biology that from the start confined women to a constant round of childbearing and caring, giving men their chance to exclude them first from the hunting pack, then from the councils of power, and in that way, from access to wealth and influence in their own right.

In our Western culture that, now, is changing. If we wish to use it, today we have the power to control the biology that once controlled us.

This comes not only in the form of effective contraception that allows us to limit our families and combine 'wanted' children with jobs and careers, if we wish or need to do this. Biological Lib comes also through the choice we now have in terms of menopause, that second brake that nature applied to female energies and enterprise. With replacement therapy available it's no longer necessary to undergo the adverse effects of hormone deficiency or live a third of our lives without the hormones that preserve both our physical and mental capacities and wellbeing.

Loss of the ovarian hormones can often bring psychological problems as severe and damaging as the physical ones. So on top of the usual flushes, night sweats, vaginal atrophy, loss of energy and loss of libido, many women also have to cope with loss of memory and confidence, confusion, inability to make decisions, and bouts of irrational irritability and depression.

In an extensive survey of women's attitudes to the menopause, carried out by the International Health Foundation in five European countries, these mental symptoms were found to be the ones women worried about and complained about most, simply because they so often spilled over to affect their relationships and efficiency both at home and at work.

If they are severe enough, the mental effects of the menopause can certainly spell disaster for the career woman. At the age when more responsible and better-paid jobs are in the offing she may well feel unable to cope.

This emerged very clearly in the letters I received in the early days, when HRT was just coming in. Many were from career women, desperate because with the onset of menopause they felt incompetent and unable to accept promotion, or in some cases even to continue in jobs they had previously done well and happily.

The logical use of hormone therapy today makes the menopause and all its miseries obsolete. Replacing the missing oestrogen eliminates the physical and psychological symptoms, releasing the unfair brake that hormone deficiency applies to our energies and enterprise and slowing down the degenerative changes it brings, including the most dangerous of all – accelerated bone loss.[2]

Post menopausal problems are now seen correctly for what they are: not an inevitable part of ageing, but a direct result of the hormone deficiency that follows ovarian loss or failure. Proof positive of this lies in the fact that quite young women experience exactly the same symptoms and exactly the same increased bone loss if they run into early natural or surgical menopause. As a result, they run an especially high risk of developing osteoporosis, simply because of those *extra* years during which accelerated bone loss can occur.

For these women HRT is particularly and strongly recommended.

With the concept of hormone replacement already the established and accepted treatment for *other* hormone deficiency states such as thyroid, adrenal or diabetes, it was always a short logical step for the same principle to be extended to the adverse effects of the menopause. And it has proved to be just as successful.

Press and media reports often given the impression that using HRT to treat menopause problems, including prevention of bone loss, is something new and controversial. It has actually been around for a long time, though not widely used. But even in this country there are some examples of women lucky enough to have had forward-looking doctors as long ago as the fifties. Lucy Fields is one of them. She was put on HRT thirty years ago because her own mother had died as a result of osteoporosis, known in those days, as 'decalcification'. Lucy is now seventy-eight and a recent scan showed she had the bones of a fifty year old. She is a wonderful example of the benefits of long-term therapy and, needless to say, is a keen supporter of the National Osteoporosis Society and of HRT.

My book, *No Change*, traces the use of HRT for more than a quarter of a century, up to the present day, and details the modern research and refinements that have now made it so easy for GPs to prescribe and so safe for patients to use.

Despite these advances and the space devoted to them in the medical journals, however, it has taken fifteen years to overcome the conditioning that generated initial resistance to HRT among doctors in the UK. Even now, when there is irrefutable evidence of the benefits of HRT and when it is increasingly widely available through GPs, gynaecological departments and menopause clinics, there are still a few family doctors who remain obstinately blinkered, refusing to prescribe it and often giving no explanation for their attitude – or worse still, one that is totally unfounded in fact.

Fortunately, when situations like this occur today there are ways around what was once an almost insoluble situation. Chapter Five explains how to set about getting this treatment if your own GP should be less than helpful. It also explains the balance of risk and benefit, lists the few contra-indications, the even fewer side-effects, and describes the different modern methods of administration, comparing their separate advantages and disadvantages. In addition, this chapter outlines some of the many studies which have confirmed that HRT given early both prevents post-menopausal bone loss and reduces the risk of fractures.

Quite apart from loss of protective oestrogen at the menopause, there are other adverse factors that can affect our bones over the years. Many of them are linked to our lifestyle, and there are appropriate strategies that can be adopted to combat them. But before we go into detail about both the positive and negative influences that can affect bone density, and before we look at how our own individual risk of osteoporosis can be assessed and dealt with, it's necessary first to know a little about bone itself. It's by no means the solid, dull, inert substance it appears to be, but rather it's a complex living tissue with a variety of fascinating and vital tasks to perform.

Chapter 2
Living bone

Most of us probably think of bone as inert and static because that's the way we normally see it – just lifeless chunks lying around the butcher's shop or desiccated remains dug up by the dog.

But in the living body, bone is living tissue, richly supplied with blood vessels, nerve fibres and fluid-filled channels, ready to perform complex tasks. Almost everything that happens to us can affect our bone and certainly everything that happens to our bone affects us.

Versatile bone

Of course, the most obvious function of the 206 bones contained in the human body is to give it shape and strength. Without it we should be as floppy as jelly-fish.

But bone does much more than form a framework for muscle and flesh. It also manufactures vital blood cells and stores ninety-nine per cent of the body's highly essential calcium supplies. This acts as an emergency reserve on which the body can draw, if and when the precise balance of calcium required in the blood needs to be topped up.

The remaining one per cent of calcium contained in blood, soft tissues and fluids throughout the body has to be kept at an exactly constant level if muscle contractions (including those of the heart) are to be kept working properly, and normal blood clotting and brain function is to be ensured. This function of calcium is so imperative that if it's necessary to make up any deficit, a powerful hormone control system goes into immediate action in our bodies actually to leach calcium from our own bones.

Such periodic raids on bone mass can take place for a variety of reasons. A common one is when anyone slims so obsessively that her diet becomes severely lacking in calcium, and there are many studies showing osteoporosis developing following anorexia, with loss of periods (indicating loss of oestrogen).[1]

Of course, calcium starvation also occurs – more sadly, more unavoidably and far more often – in the Third World as a result of poverty and famine. As usual, it is the women who suffer most during food shortages, both because they give their own meagre rations to their children to try to keep them alive, and because pregnancy makes special demands. A baby in the womb always has first call on nutrients including limited calcium supplies needed for its own developing bones. This commonly means that the price poorly nourished women pay for motherhood is porous weakened bones and lost teeth.

How new bone is made

With all of us, under ordinary circumstances, a constant turnover of bone still takes place, with old bone being broken down and new bone formed. This normal cycle of resorption and renewal is common to all living tissues.

The balance of bone in our bodies varies at different periods of our lives. In the early years, obviously, more bone has to be laid down than is resorbed, to allow for growth. The spectacular growth spurt of puberty creates an especially heavy demand for new bone. Fortunately the surge of sex hormones that produce sexual maturity also stimulate the required extra bone formation.

Throughout life there is always the need for a certain amount of new bone to repair the minascule fractures that result from day-to-day wear and tear and to replace bone that would otherwise get worn out.

Special 'demolition' gangs of cells called 'osteoclasts' are responsible for starting the turnover process by digging minute cavities along the inner surface of the bone. Following that, even larger gangs of 'builder' cells knows as 'osteoblasts' take over, filling in the cavities with new bone cells, around which protein fibres (made up primarily of collagen) form.

After about ten days, crystals of calcium and phosphate are laid down, embedding themselves in the interlocking collagen fibres. While the collagen content gives bone the limited flexibility it has, the mineral content gives it hardness, rigidity and strength.

Small quantities of other materials such as fluoride, sodium potassium, magnesium and citrate are also present in bone, together with a few other trace elements, all acting as mortar to hold together the 'bricks' of calcium and phosphate crystals.

This bone 'mineralization' process takes from several weeks to a few months to complete and the entire cycle lasts approximately three to four months. It's estimated adults may have between ten to thirty per cent of their bone replaced each year in this way.

The changing balance

Not long after puberty, the balance starts to change and even in our early thirties slightly more bone is resorbed than is laid down, so that over the years our skeletal structure gradually weakens. Bones don't decrease in size or radius, of course, but become less dense. This age-related loss that makes bones more porous occurs in both sexes, though to a much lesser degree in men than in women.

Awareness of this progressive bone loss should make all of us, even as young adults, take positive steps to minimize the effect and preserve as healthy and strong a bone mass as possible. A well-balanced diet with adequate calcium intake helps, as does taking the regular exercise which is so vital to bone retention. Chapter six goes into greater detail about diet and exercise, and other strategies, such as avoiding substances that act as bone robbers.

These bone robbers include some conventional medical drugs, such as cortisone, which have the side-effect of depleting bone. When no other effective treatment is available, some drugs may well have to be taken, and under those circumstances, a good doctor will take into account the adverse effect on bone and prescribe with caution, keeping the courses as short as possible and perhaps also advising calcium supplementation.

For now we need to understand a bit more about bone itself and *why* certain areas are so vulnerable to the thinning process that they form common sites for osteoporotic fracture.

High-risk bones

There are actually two quite different types of bone in our bodies. There is the outer cortical bone which is solid and dense, and the inner trabecular bone which looks rather like honeycomb or an Aero chocolate bar. Although the trabecular bone structure provides a light and surprisingly strong framework, it also allows a greater surface area than cortical bone upon which the osteoclasts can work – and therefore for the bone eroding process to take place (Figure 1).

As a result, areas with a higher proportion of

Vertebra (back bone)

Femur (thigh bone)

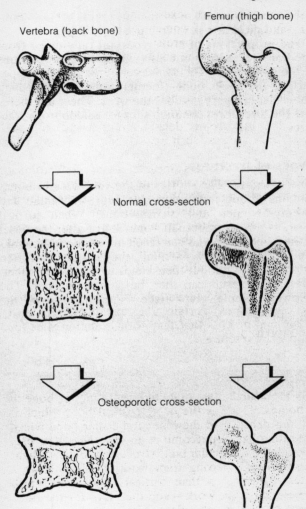

Normal cross-section

Osteoporotic cross-section

Figure 1 Bone-eroding process

trabecular bone tend to be the most vulnerable to thinning and most at risk of fracture.

The proportions of both types not only differ from one bone to another but also within different sections of the *same* bone. The spinal vertebrae and the upper part of the thigh bone (femur) come into the high trabecular category, as does the wrist. These are therefore the three most common sites for osteoporotic fractures.

Types of fractures

Wrist fractures: The shorter of the two forearm bones contains about twenty-five per cent trabecular and seventy-five per cent cortical bone. When cortical bone, as well as trabecular bone, is lost after the onset of the menopause, this can result in considerably weakened wrists. When women fall, they commonly (often automatically) put out their hands to try to save themselves. The result can then be a broken wrist. The following simple graph (see Figure 2) shows the

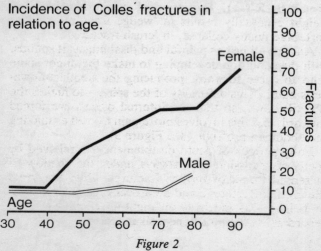

Figure 2

amazing tenfold rise in this type of fracture (called a Colles' fracture) in women over the age of fifty. The other line on the graph shows no comparable rise for men.

Spinal fractures: The body of each vertebra is made up of ninety per cent trabecular bone. As this is lost at an increased rate following the menopause and because the remaining cortical shell also becomes thinner, the weight of the body can sometimes become too much for the spine to bear. The average age when the resulting spinal deformity or fracture tends to show up is sixty, but it can happen any time between the ages of fifty and seventy. Much depends on how early the menopause and the consequent bone loss started to occur, together with the *rate* at which it takes place.

The usual course of events is that as the vertebrae become more porous and weak, they gradually change from a rectangular to a wedge shape. Half of all women at sixty-five who have *not* been protected by HRT, show detectable 'wedging', as it's called (this is confirmed by X-ray). The strain of supporting the body weight eventually results in 'wedge fractures' and as vertebrae finally collapse, in 'crush fractures'.

And it's all just as painful and disabling as it sounds, with the condition developing to make the upper spine tend to curve forward, producing the familiar dowager's hump. This deformity of the spine also makes the ribs tilt down, so that the internal organs are forced forward, and this involves more pain as well as making the abdomen protrude (see Figure 3).

Long periods of acute disablement are relieved by spells of remission, but always under the shadow of increased threat of further fractures. Over the years the crushed vertebrae and bent backs rob their victims of height – as much as an eight-inch loss has been recorded in severe osteoporosis cases.

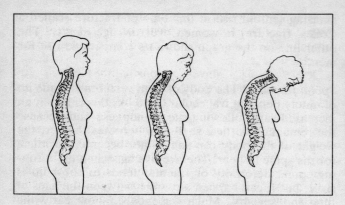

Figure 3 Formation of a dowager's hump

When Joan Lister, a fifty-one-year-old nurse, developed severe low back pain after doing some heavy lifting it was presumed to be a strained back. Neither she nor her GP picked up the warning signs of spinal osteoporosis and she suffered four crush fractures, lost three inches in height and fifty per cent of her bone mineral density before the problem was correctly diagnosed.

Joan was away from her job for a month with her first bout of pain and only two months after returning to nursing she encountered a second and more severe episode. This time the pain was so acute that it was increased by the slightest movement, even coughing. After yet another month at home the condition eased somewhat, but there was no way she could return to a job which inevitably involved lifting.

It was then that Joan's GP referred her to an osteopath who had an X-ray taken; this revealed nothing. Treatment was started that only made matters worse. Things were so bad that Joan couldn't even lie prone for spinal manipulation. A second X-ray was done.

This time collapsed vertebrae showed up, so at that point, after three months mostly off work and mostly in pain, she was at last referred to an appropriate specialist.

The specialists' investigations confirmed the full extent of the osteoporotic damage, and the case history he took pinpointed several known high risk factors that would have contributed to such early and heavy bone loss – there was the fact that Joan had ceased to menstruate at only forty-three, imposing extra years of accelerated bone loss as a result of early natural menopause; the fact that she was thin and of light build, with a relatively light bone mass to withstand the menopausal onslaught; and, finally, she had never taken regular exercise and had smoked ten cigarettes a day for over twenty years.

Because Joan had never suffered flushes, night sweats or any of the obvious menopausal symptoms, she'd not felt the need to consult her doctor when menstruation ceased early. Despite being a nurse she had not realized that premature menopause puts a woman at especial risk of brittle bones. Because lack of knowledge about osteoporosis prevented the necessary treatment, the damage was done before appropriate action could be taken; damage that could not be reversed.

In Joan's case specialist investigation uncovered another factor that had contributed to her condition. 'Our investigations showed this patient also suffered from an over-active thyroid gland', her specialist told me. 'This condition also adversely affects bone mass and this discovery confirms the usefulness of screening post-menopausal women with osteoporosis for disorders not linked to the menopause but that also affect bone.'

Joan is now on medication to combat the over-active thyroid, and undergoing Hormone Replacement Therapy to counter post-menopausal oestrogen deficiency. Both will help to some degree, but there is little chance of her returning to nursing or a fully normal, active life.

I am deliberately not pulling any punches in describing the miserable consequences of osteoporosis, because, distressing enough in themselves, they are doubly so when you consider that they don't need to happen.

In ninety-nine per cent of instances, osteoporotic fractures could have been prevented if correct protective action had been taken and HRT used early enough. This is now accepted by the medical establishment, as the Consensus Development Conference at Aalborg, and a 1989 report from the College of Physicians on hip fractures both confirm. This puts responsibility firmly with doctors, but women themselves also have a part to play in seeing that the necessary action is taken and *unnecessary* suffering avoided.

Hip fractures: Because the neck of the femur has a higher proportion of cortical bone than the spine (fifty per cent trabecular and fifty per cent cortical), women tend to run into hip fractures rather later than spinal fractures. But from the mid-seventies the point can be reached when a great deal of trabecular bone has been lost and outer cortical bone has also become very thin. From then on, a fall which normal bone could withstand may cause the now porous narrow neck of the femur to snap. (See Figure 4)

The sort of accident that results in this common hip fracture often occurs when getting in or out of the bath or by merely tripping on uneven pavements or rugs. Occasionally, however, hip fractures happen quite spontaneously – simply because the vital area of bone

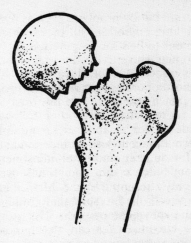

Figure 4 Location of hip fracture

has become too fragile to bear the transfer of weight from one leg to another, even briefly, as a step is taken. Of course, when the hip breaks a fall follows, and there can often be some confusion about which came first.

As the 1989 report from the Royal College of Physicians emphasizes, we are currently in the middle of a positive 'epidemic' of hip fractures in elderly women. Many hospitals are so overloaded with patients that transfer to the operating theatre is delayed, and thus treatment is often far from satisfactory. This situation is likely to get worse until the number of these fractures can be drastically reduced by taking the advice of Sir Raymond Hoffenberg, who, as president of the Royal College, urged all women to consider HRT to prevent their bones becoming so dangerously weak.

Hip fractures are certainly the most dangerous and life-threatening of all osteoporotic fractures, carrying a death rate of one in six.[2] Death is seldom caused by the actual fracture but by problems such as pneumonia, thrombosis or lung embolism, all of which can result from confinement to bed for long periods.

Even for women who survive the trauma and immobilization, the effects can be devastating. The most cruel aspect of osteoporosis is its relentless progression. Studies have shown that after one hip break, there is twenty times more risk of the other following. The increased tendency for disabilities to multiply brings not only deformation but loss of independence, both of which call for difficult emotional adjustment.

Loss of independence can sometimes occur quite early and not only after hip fracture. Mrs Lilian Lolley, sixty-five, has already had to seek sheltered housing as a result of acute spinal osteoporosis. Her story vividly illustrates how circumstances can cruelly combine to suddenly impose heavy bone loss that results in osteoporosis unless it is countered.

At only forty-two, Lilian had been diagnosed as having severe rheumatoid arthritis and she had been put on corticosteroids, notorious bone robbers but essential for the management of this condition. At that time her ovarian function was still normal, but by forty-five her periods had become irregular and at forty-seven menstruation ceased completely. At a relatively young age this woman, who had no family history of osteoporosis and who had always taken exercise and never smoked, ran into two bone depleting conditions – the absolute need for steroid drugs for which there was no real substitute, and the onset of a somewhat early menopause with loss of protective oestrogen.

From then on the real tragedy lay in the total failure of her doctors to foresee her increased risk of osteoporosis, or if they did foresee it to do anything to circumvent or limit it. Even if, back in the seventies, her GP might not yet have been fully familiar with the situation, her rheumatologist certainly should have

been. In fact he not only seemed ignorant of the need
to do anything special to protect her against the effects
of the steroid treatment he was forced to prescribe,
but in 1982 he ignored her complaints of very severe
back pain on bending and of the acute and terrible
agony she experienced on one occasion when she
chanced to cough and sneeze at the same time. In
both cases he dismissed the symptoms as 'only to be
expected and just part of your arthritis'.

Of course, they were nothing of the sort. They were
severe, established osteoporosis making itself felt.
When she did finally achieve referral to the Royal
National Hospital at Bath a year later, X-rays showed
two severe vertebral fractures just two inches from the
base of the spine.

It was through reading an article in *Arthritis Care*
magazine that Lilian realized the possible serious
nature of her problem, and through an allied arthritis
charity that she got the vital advice to seek referral to
the specialist hospital at Bath.

And even that did not prove easy: her GP insisted
it was all quite unnecessary as she was already in the
best hands. He told her he would give her no help with
transport and she would have to get there under her
own steam. Only with great reluctance did he finally
yield the referral letter necessary for the consultation.

So it was not until 1983, when the severe and irreversible osteoporotic damage had already taken place,
that Lilian finally reached a real source of expert diagnosis and treatment – and that was the result of her
own enterprise and determination.

Investigation showed two spinal fractures and a loss
of seven and a half inches in height, with a very pro-
nounced dowager's hump and, in consequence, ribs
pushed forward and down below the pelvis. Only special exercises, initiated by Dr Allan Dixon, which
Lilian has to maintain, enable her to hold her head up

and avoid the total bent-over stance typical of many women with acute spinal osteoporosis.

Hers is a story of great courage and a great fight to maintain independence. Put on HRT, supplemented by calcium and fluoride tablets, and with periods of in-patient treatment at the Royal National Hospital in Bath, Lilian and her husband struggled until 1986 to keep their own home. By then, with only one and a half hours official home help allowed in the part of Dorset where they were then living, it became clear they could not go on any longer.

Through Help The Aged, the Lolleys were finally rehoused in a flat in a residential home in Bristol, where they could be together, with an SRN always on duty, special ramps and facilities and the main meal supplied each day. It's not independence and it's not like being in their own home, but Lilian is grateful for it and she is comfortingly near the Bath Hospital where her condition continues to be supervised and managed.

'I shall always be grateful to them and to the National Osteoporosis Society which does so much to help people like me,' Lilian told me. 'I have gone on television for them and am happy for my case to go into your book, in the hope that it may help other women to avoid the pain I have to endure. I also hope it may alert doctors to make them more aware of special risk factors and of early symptoms of osteoporosis so that preventive measures can be taken in time.'

Where disease or disaster are concerned we often talk about prevention being better than cure, but with osteoporosis there *is* no cure and prevention is the one real hope.

In the present state of knowledge, only in a very few instances can bone already lost ever be restored. But fortunately it's never too late to start HRT. Even some years into the menopause, replacing the missing hormones will cut back on further heavy bone loss, and even after an initial Colles' fracture has given the first warning, HRT can help to prevent further fractures.[3] It seems that the old saying 'Better late than never' is the one that applies in this case. In fact, getting on to HRT as quickly as possible is vital where the onset of osteoporosis is diagnosed or high risk of its developing suspected.

Just how you and your doctor can assess *your* individual likelihood of developing osteoporosis is discussed in the next chapter. But because complex hormonal factors play such a big part in this, I'll explain how it's thought hormones act and interact to affect bone growth and bone loss. It's a pretty complex theory, so if you really can't be bothered with a lot of detail don't worry – just skip to the summary at the end of this chapter.

Hormones and bone

Growth hormone: This hormone, produced by the pituitary gland, is responsible for triggering initial growth in many tissues, including bone. Experts believe that where bone is concerned growth hormone works by stimulating the two gangs of cells involved in the formation and resorption of bone. Research into this theory and how it may be affected by the menopause is continuing. Early research suggests that women who develop osteoporosis after the menopause produce less growth hormone than those who don't have this problem but there is much more work to be done.

Thyroid hormones: These come from the thyroid gland in the neck and are also vital for proper formation of bone mass in the early years. Deficiency at that stage again results in stunted development, while excess at any time in our lives can *over*-stimulate the bone turn-over process and cause excessive bone loss, as Joan Lister's case history shows. Modern treatments can correct both hyperthyroidism (over-production) and hypothyroidism (under-production) of thyroid hormone.

Parathyroid hormone: This is produced from four little glands in the neck at the back of the thyroid gland, and acts to increase the level of calcium in the blood. If and when this falls too low, the parathyroid hormone is released into the bloodstream, and this causes the kidneys to excrete phosphate. To compensate for this, phosphate is taken from the bones bringing calcium with it.

Parathyroid also stimulates the conversion of Vitamin D from an inactive form to an active form able to encourage the intestines to absorb more calcium from food.

Its third mechanism is to stimulate the breakdown of bone, so that calcium stores are released into the bloodstream.

Vitamin D: Don't be surprised to see Vitamin D listed in the hormone section as these days it's more properly considered a hormone than a vitamin.

Vitamin D is produced by the effect of sunshine on the skin and also comes from foods such as milk, fish and eggs. Stored in the liver as an *inactive* substance, conversion to the active form takes place in the kidneys, after which it's able to increase the resorption of calcium.

Very like parathyroid hormone, Vitamin D maintains the calcium – phosphate levels in the bloodstream and again, like parathyroid hormone, if present at too high a level it actually extracts calcium from the bone.

It's important to remember this, particularly when taking it as a vitamin supplement.

Calcitonin: This is another hormone released mainly by the thyroid gland. It is known as a 'calcium-sparing' hormone because it helps to protect against the adverse effects of parathyroid hormone and Vitamin D when these seek to rob us of bone. Exactly how it works is not yet completely understood, but it's thought to slow down the activity of the osteoclasts, the cells whose job it is to break down bone.

Calcitonin levels decrease with age, and this may be one of the reasons we all lose bone as we get older. It's also known that men have more of this hormone than women, and that women who *don't* develop osteoporosis have more calcitonin than women who do. So, however it actually works, there's evidence that calcitonin plays an important protective role.

Adrenal hormones: In response to physical or emotional stress and danger, the adrenal glands, situated near the kidneys, send out great surges of adrenaline hormones into the bloodstream. These prepare the body for action, triggering what is often called the 'fight or flight' mechanism.

Clearly, adrenaline has always been and still is vital to our survival, but as with other powerful hormones there can be a negative side, which tends to come into operation if the output is not correctly balanced.

In this case, *over*-activity of the adrenal gland is associated with severe osteoporosis, as is long-term use of drugs (such as hydrocortisone) that resemble the adrenal hormones. Both interact with the parathyroid hormone and Vitamin D to dissolve bone. If this process went unchecked terrible damage to our bones would result, but fortunately the female sex hormones

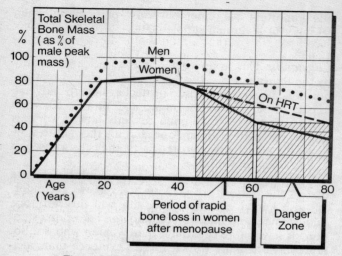

Figure 5 Changes in bone mass with age

also interact with the adrenal hormones and limit their adverse effect.

After the menopause the control exerted by the sex hormones is diminished and therefore a great deal of bone is lost for about the next fifteen years. Then, at around sixty-five our adrenal glands slow down production and that is assumed to be why the rate of bone loss begins to drop around that age (see Figure 5).

Oestrogen and progesterone: In pre-menopause days oestrogen comes to the rescue of bone in women by stimulating the liver to produce a protein that reduces the ability of the adrenal hormones to dissolve bone. Inhibiting adrenal action is not the only way in which oestrogen helps protect bone. It also blocks the harmful action of the parathyroid hormone on bone mass.

Finally, it stimulates Vitamin D and calcitonin to carry out their special bone-protecting functions. Studies have confirmed this action both during pregnancy (when oestrogen levels are high) *and* when oestrogen is prescribed by HRT after the menopause[4]. When oestrogen production ceases, all such benefits also cease and, unless replacement therapy is used, drastically accelerated bone loss takes place.

Progesterone, the female hormone produced by the ovaries in the second half of the menstrual cycle, appears also to aid bone protection by similarly helping to inhibit the action of the adrenal hormones.

The information you've just read is the most difficult we have to deal with in learning about osteoporosis. By comparison the rest is simple and straightforward. In the next chapter we can now look at all the different factors that affect bone mass and need to be taken into consideration when assessing our individual risk of developing osteoporosis.

Meanwhile, here is a brief summary that may help clarify the hormonal influences it could be useful to remember, particularly in relation to oestrogen and progestrone protection:

Hormone influences on bone mass

Helpful	*Harmful*
Growth hormone from pituitary	Deficiency of growth hormone
Calcitonin from the thyroid	Excessive activity of thyroid
Vitamin D from liver and kidneys	Excessive activity of adrenocortical hormones

Helpful	*Harmful*
Oestrogen and progesterone from ovaries (in women)	Deficiency of oestrogen and progesterone
Testosterone from testes (in men)	

Chapter 3

Assessing *your* risk of osteoporosis

It's never possible to predict with absolute certainty your chances of suffering from osteoporosis. There are, however, a whole lot of factors which are known to either increase or diminish the likelihood of developing it, and which should be taken into account when trying to determine if you are going to be in the low, average or high-risk category.

Some of the factors affecting osteoporosis risks (for better or for worse) fall within *your* control, and later in the book you will find details of the positive steps you can take to minimize bone loss and keep osteoporosis at bay.

In contrast, however, there are other influences, already pre-determined and about which you can usually do nothing, *except* make sure they are included on the appropriate plus or minus side of the final equation used to estimate your potential osteoporosis status. It's usually a good idea to enlist the help of your GP or gynaecologist in doing this, so that together you can decide just what protective measures are required in your particular case and how important it is for them to be taken early.

The pre-determined factors

For the most part the influences you can do nothing about are the ones dictated by genes and heredity. Gender, racial origins, inherited characteristics relating to skeletal mass and any history of osteoporosis in the family can all have bearing on subsequent osteoporosis risk, and there is no element of choice in these matters. We are stuck with them as part of the lottery of conception and birth – the biggest gamble of our lives.

Gender: We've already looked briefly at 'the female factor' and found that simply being born a woman puts us straight into the front line in the battle against osteoporosis. In this chapter we'll be looking more fully at the implications of being female, but this time from the point of view of assessing *your* individual risk. There are so many things that can happen to a woman's body during her life (which just can't happen to a man's) and many of them can influence her chances of developing brittle bones one way or another.

For example, being on the combined contraceptive pill or having babies can be positively helpful in *slowing down* the bone-thinning process, as both involve raised oestrogen levels, with associated increased protection against bone loss, over the actual pregnancy and breastfeeding periods or during the years of oral contraceptive use.

Racial influences: It seems far stranger that race should enter into this particular risk equation. But the reason for this is that women of African, Aboriginal or even Mediterranean origin seem in general to have thicker bones and a greater bone mass at skeletal maturity than do white Caucasian or Oriental women. They also on average have bigger muscles that exert greater stress and pull on the bones – something already noted as being helpful in maintaining density and strength of bones.

In addition such women also seem to lose bone more slowly than white females as they get older. This can probably be explained by hormonal differences, in particular by the higher levels of calcitonin which scientific tests have shown they possess. All these advantages taken together help to explain why so many studies have confirmed less osteoporosis in these races – in fact, the condition is almost unknown in African women.

However African and Asian females do develop osteoporosis when they live for long periods in northern latitudes. Dark skin pigmentation can be a distinct disadvantage when living under weaker or more fitful sun, as it presents too great a barrier to the ultra-violet light required to manufacture adequate amounts of Vitamin D in the body. Less Vitamin D, as we have seen, in turn means less absorption of calcium.

Family history: Apart from genetic influences at work within different races, there are also genetic influences at work within different families. A predisposition towards osteoporosis can be inherited from either the mother's or the father's side. Highly relevant factors such as the amount of bone mass you're likely to have at skeletal maturity and the rate at which bone is lost with age appear to be among genetically determined characteristics.

Strong evidence for this comes from studies of twins. Identical twins (coming from a single egg dividing) have been shown to possess more closely matched bone mass than fraternal twins (coming from two separate eggs) and both types tend to have more closely matched bone mass than ordinary siblings.[1] Doctors have confirmed that many (though by no means *all*) women with osteoporosis, have a history of this disorder in their families.

Pamela Halstead's story shows how osteoporosis can suddenly interrupt a career, and even force early retirement. As a deputy head, Pam loved her job of teaching very small children. Then, when she was only fifty, she began to experience terrible low-back pain. X-rays revealed osteoporosis and some osteo-arthritis. Her GP simply prescribed calcium and it was some time before she managed to contact the National Osteoporosis Society and get referred to a specialist. More X-rays confirmed the condition and she was immediately put on HRT, but by then the pain was so excruciating that she had no option but to take early retirement on medical grounds.

Pam told me, 'I have very small bones and my mother was exactly the same. I remember her when she was only in her sixties leaning over the side of the sofa to pick up her knitting. The sofa arms were soft but the pressure on her ribs was still enough to crack two of them. She died soon after so I never saw the condition progress. But I just wish I'd known more about osteoporosis earlier, so that I might have realized I was at high risk myself. I feel then I would at least have had a choice to try and protect myself before the damage was done.'

Pamela's family history indicates a high osteoporosis risk.

So, an indicator of your own possible risk of getting osteoporosis can be seeing how other females in your family have fared in this respect, particularly your mother, sisters, grandmothers or even aunts or great aunts. If any of them have suffered from brittle bone problems (showing up perhaps as fractures or shrinkage in height with ageing) then *you* should accept that you probably come from a high-risk family.

But don't let it worry you. It's useful to know because these days, fortunately, there's plenty you can do to prevent a similar fate overtaking you. As you near the menopause it becomes especially important to let your GP know if a family background of osteoporosis seems to exist, so that the importance of putting you on HRT in good time is understood. Few GPs who know their job will argue about such a wise precaution at that point. Until then you should, of course, be taking all the self-help measures that assist in building and protecting your bone mass.

Unfortunately, although finding no family history of the disease is encouraging and has to be good news, it doesn't absolutely ensure that you're in the clear yourself. Other *non*-hereditary factors, described below, can be involved and change the picture.

There is further good news (rather surprisingly) if you tend to plumpness. While inheriting small bones and/or slim stature *add* to the chances of developing osteoporosis, inheriting a tendency to be well covered actually *decreases* them. This is partly because extra weight puts extra beneficial stress on the bones, but more importantly because fatty tissue also allows conversion of substances called oestrogen precursors into actual oestrogen after the menopause.

Oestrogen precursors in the form of very small amounts of male hormones are produced by the ovaries long after they have ceased to yield much in the way of female hormones. The adrenal glands produce much more male hormone, but from both sources the vital transformation into protective oestrogen can only take place in fatty tissue. So from the health angle (for once) a bit of fat positively pays off. The extra oestrogen being naturally manufactured in the body in this way also brings cosmetic advantage and is the reason why so many plump women retain good creamy skins, smoother and less prone to wrinkles than in the rest of us. They also, of course, tend to experience relatively fewer menopause symptoms – in a few cases even none at all!

Age of menopause: The presence of oestrogen, as

we've seen, is the key factor in preventing the increased bone loss that otherwise leads eventually to osteoporosis in far too many women. It follows logically that the *later* the menopause occurs, the longer your bones continue to benefit from this basic hormone protection.

The age of menopause is again something that in the main you can do little about. As we've seen it's part of the female blueprint and consequently pre-determined by your inherited genetic makeup. This shows clearly in the close link so often found in the age of menopause in mothers and daughters. This is most clearly highlighted in cases of early-menopause families. Researching for my book, *No Change*, I came across one family where the mother ceased to menstruate at forty-two and her three daughters at thirty-three, thirty-three and thirty-eight respectively. So, if *you* find early menopause tends to run in *your* family, there is a distinct possibility your own ovaries may also be programmed to pack up early. In such cases it's a good idea to be prepared and ready to offset the adverse effect on bone mass by adopting in advance a regime of an adequate calcium diet and exercise – not to mention, of course, prompt resort to HRT when the time comes.

Someone who took very determined action to get HRT protection in exactly that situation was Christine Roberts. Her own mother had started what proved to be a truly terrible menopause at the age of only thirtynine. The irritability and depression it produced were so severe that they spilled over to affect the whole family. In time, her mother became a tragic victim of osteoporosis and in a recent fall broke her arm and shoulder, as well as cracking her ribs.

Ominously, Christine started the menopause at a similar age, just five days after her fortieth birthday. The pattern seemed to be repeating itself with eighteen months of depression, night sweats and other miseries

very like those her mother experienced. After reading
No Change she made repeated efforts to get HRT
from any of the six doctors in the group practice she
attended. But only when she finally threatened to go
privately if they continued to refuse a trial course of
HRT, did she finally win the day and get treatment.
She wrote to tell me that it has been a great success
and within two months the symptoms had cleared. In
the longer term, she now feels confident that she will
also be protected against the problems of brittle and
broken bones that have beset her mother.

In **Women's Views and Statements**, page 130
Christine tells how these same GPs first argued that
she was too young to be undergoing the 'change'.
When they finally admitted she was indeed suffering
menopause, they insisted that HRT wouldn't help
natural menopausal symptoms. They told her to put
up with it! If some doctors do still try to insist that the
menopause is natural – they can hardly make the same
claim for brittle and broken bones!

Non genetic reasons for premature menopause

Smoking: Although the mechanism at work is not fully
understood, numerous studies have proved beyond
doubt that smoking adversely affects hormone levels
and precipitates a premature menopause.[2] This is one
of the controllable factors that you *can* do something
about. If you smoke it's really worth trying to kick a
habit that's as hard on your pocket as it is on your
health. Giving up smoking will not only protect against
lung and cervical cancer, not to mention bronchial and
heart problems, but also help to avoid crumbling
broken bones and the pain and disfigurement of osteoporosis.

If you want even more encouragement, remember

that the lower oestrogen levels that result from smoking also inflict premature ageing in the form of earlier and deeper wrinkling and drying of the skin, as well as the drying and shrinkage of the vagina (vaginal atrophy) which can ruin your sex life and hazard sexual relationships. Topping up oestrogen levels via HRT at the menopause would seem to offer an easy way out: it compensates for the lower oestrogen levels caused by smoking and slows down related aspects of ageing, with excellent cosmetic effects on skin and hair, as well as keeping bones healthy and the vagina elastic and lubricated. But there can be a Catch-22 situation for smokers. Some GPs do not like prescribing HRT for women who smoke heavily and refuse to give it up when asking for replacement therapy. This is an over-cautious reaction on the doctor's part, but it can still make getting the treatment that much more difficult. The chapter on HRT will explain *why* fears about smoking and HRT still sometimes mistakenly persist.

Alcohol: While on the subject of bad habits that can affect bone mass and increase risk of osteoporosis, it's a good time to make the point that many studies have shown heavy drinkers to have abnormally light bones. This is partly due to the fact that alcohol in quantity affects the ability of the liver to activate Vitamin D (important in calcium absorption) and therefore impairs calcium absorption through the intestines. To be honest, it's not known if moderate amounts of alcohol also have similar adverse effects but it does fall into the bone-robber class. After that it's up to you and your estimated general osteoporosis risk to decide how closely you should discipline your alcohol intake.

Hysterectomy (surgical removal of womb): Hysterectomy is rarely within your control; if recommended by a gynaecologist, it is usually unavoidable. Unfortunately it's again something recognized as an induction factor in early menopause. Where there is *real* medical justification for removing the womb, of course there is no question of trying to avoid this surgery, and in such cases it almost invariably confers enormous benefit. These days, it is also a very safe operation. Nevertheless, it's worthwhile making quite sure that your gynaecologist has no other option in dealing with your problem.

I know from my American research that over there wombs are certainly removed far too freely, often it seems more to protect the doctor against possible future litigation problems than to protect the woman against possible future health problems. This doesn't happen to the same extent in this country, where NHS restrictions hardly encourage unnecessary surgery, but it's still worth making quite sure your hysterectomy really is necessary, as the records show that within two years of this surgery's being carried out the ovaries begin to fail even in quite young women[3] in one case in four.

This premature onset of the menopause happens despite surgery being restricted to the womb, leaving the ovaries untouched (simple hysterectomy). Leaving even one ovary or just half an ovary should logically enable enough oestrogen to be produced to keep the menopause at bay until the normal age for ovarian failure (on average around fifty). The reason for premature ovarian shutdown being precipitated – after a quarter of all hysterectomies – is believed to be because the operation interferes with the blood supply to the ovaries and makes them become less efficient or, as some experts suggest, because removal of the womb in some subtle way discourages hormone production.

Whatever the reason, the result is the same, and regardless of age any woman who has had her womb removed should not hesitate to consult her GP or gynaecologist if she starts to experience flushes, vaginal atrophy, palpitations, unnatural tiredness, depression or any of the other typical overt menopause symptoms. Even if she bravely feels she can cope with these more obvious problems, she should remember that the 'silent' effect of bone disintegration will also have started bringing with it an above-average risk of developing osteoporosis because of the extra years of increased bone loss. Happily, HRT adopted in good time not only prevents all this but is particularly simple for the woman without a womb. In such a case HRT can be based on use of just oestrogen and this allows all the usual advantages of renewed energy, improved libido, vital bone protection, elimination of flushes, etc., *without* the disadvantage of an obligatory monthly bleed, the price that other women have to pay for modern protection against uterine cancer. This is all explained fully in Chapter Five.

One word of warning: If you are well below normal menopause age when you have your hysterectomy and your ovaries have been retained or if you run into a rather early natural menopause, it's not easy to convince some GPs that you really are entering the climacteric. If so, there is a simple and painless blood test available which you can ask to have done. This measures the level of Follicle Stimulating Hormone (FSH) in the blood. If the ovaries really are starting to fail or have already failed, then FSH levels *always* rise in an attempt to prod them back into action. Another test that often correlates even better with menopause status is a check on blood oestradiol levels. So don't be put off. If you have any difficulty in convincing your GP, insist that he or she arranges the test *or* refers you back to a gynaecologist. He or she will be familiar with many similar instances of early natural or surgical menopause among his patients.

Removal of ovaries: Of course, it goes without saying that if your gynaecologist decides that the ovaries must also be removed at the time of hysterectomy, then a surgical menopause is quite inevitable. Again it's important to discuss this and find out if this form of surgery (called an oophorectomy) is planned and, if so, if it's absolutely necessary. If there *is* any choice in the matter, then do weigh the relative pros and cons.

If your ovaries are diseased or damaged there is obviously no argument. But some gynaecologists routinely remove ovaries in older women when performing a hysterectomy on the grounds that they are also removing a possible site for future cancer. It's a valid argument, of course, but perhaps it's worth pointing out that ovarian cancer is extremely rare and is the cause of death in only one woman in 6000. By comparison removing ovaries very much prior to the natural menopause produces osteoporosis in between twenty-five and fifty women in every one hundred *unless* replacement therapy is given. And osteoporosis can be lethal, as the 6000 deaths every year of women following osteoporosis fractures of the hip makes cruelly clear. This figure has been projected to rise to 8000 by the end of 1990. A recent survey showed that in the past, seventy per cent of women who had their ovaries removed in the UK had *not* been offered HRT.[4]

This situation is changing rapidly, and it's a relief to know that most good gynaecologists performing this operation today give HRT routinely, in the form of an implant of natural oestrogen (Oestradiol) inserted at the time of surgery. Its still worth checking in advance, however, that this *is* going to be done, as it short-circuits what can otherwise be an abrupt and severe menopause. At the same time it provides the important continued hormone protection that your bones need. The first implant is either renewed when it runs out (usually after six months) or followed by a switch to

HRT given orally or via a transdermal skin patch. Either of these methods can be supervised by your GP and details about these alternative systems of administration, comparing their advantages and disadvantages, are noted in the Chapter Five.

Rate of bone loss: Second only to *age* of menopause (and thus the age at which increased bone loss starts to occur) is the *rate* of loss. As mentioned, this may well be another genetically determined factor and, therefore, a family history of osteoporosis could well indicate increased risk of *your* being among the fast bone losers.

Apart from this possible family clue, the rate of bone loss was until recently quite unpredictable. Usually the first indication of a woman's being a fast bone loser was an osteoporotic fracture. Over the last decade, however, sophisticated machines have become available that can accurately measure bone density, and readings taken some six months apart can now accurately establish the rate of loss. Details of these methods are given in Chapter Four.

Medication: There are a number of drugs either prescribed by doctors or purchased over the counter that aggravate bone loss, and some can actually cause osteoporosis to start up.

• Corticosteroids, often essential to relieve the symptoms of rheumatoid arthritis, are among the worst of the bone-robber drugs. They include cortisone-like drugs such as hydrocortisone, prednisone, prednisolone, dexamethasone and betamethasone. Their adverse effect on bone is due not only to the fact that they decrease calcium absorption and increase excretion, which is bad enough, but they also seem to act directly on bone tissue to discourage the formation of new bone. Osteoporosis induced in this way brings much more severe bone loss, as was shown by Lilian Lolley's sad case, where acute spinal osteoporosis robbed her of independence at only sixty-five.

● Anticonvulsant drugs can also cause increased bone loss by stimulating the production of enzymes that break down Vitamin D, leading to calcium deficiency.

● Antacids are often used by women for indigestion, and many of these contain aluminium which can again cause an increase in calcium excretion and contribute to bone loss. It's sensible to avoid this type. Those containing magnesium and calcium are safer.

● Diuretics must be chosen specifically for you by your doctor. Some diuretics can be dangerous calcium depleters. For example, frusemide (Lasix+K) increases urinary calcium excretion while thiazides reduce the amount of calcium lost in urine and are therefore far more appropriate for women approaching the menopause.

If you *have* to be on drugs which affect bone mass and there's no suitable alternative medication, then obviously you should discuss with your doctor what measures you can take to counter their adverse effects. It could be as simple as taking calcium supplements. The value of calcium supplements, details of calcium-rich food you can naturally include in your diet, and details of other substances best avoided in excess because they belong to the opposite group – the bone robbers – will be discussed in Chapter Six.

But for the moment let's look at the various ways doctors can test for bone loss and, in particular, the latest highly sophisticated techniques, which are becoming increasingly available and which can establish your *rate* of bone loss, a very important guide in assessing your risk status.

Chapter 4

Detecting bone loss

'Every picture tells a story' is a saying that can be cruelly apt for victims of osteoporosis, and when Margaret Harris showed me two family photographs the tale they combined to tell was all too familiar. The first was taken at her silver wedding party. Forty-eight years old then, Margaret stood beside her husband, Tom, almost as tall as he was and her figure youthful and straight. But the picture taken ten years later at the christening of one of their grandchildren made a sad contrast. Tom was as tall and straight as ever, seeming hardly to have aged in that time. But next to him, Margaret was now inches shorter and not even careful dressing could disguise the beginning of a dowager's hump.

It also proved to be the beginning of painful years of osteoporosis. In this case, as in so many, the early warning signs had been ignored. The menopause had not brought flushes severe enough for Margaret to feel she needed medical help, and Tom had been understanding about the odd moods and lack of energy which had overtaken her. Both had assumed at first that the back pain she began to experience was just temporary, and it was only when it persisted over months that she finally went to her doctor. Again, it was more months before he took the problem seriously enough to send her to a specialist.

When I met Margaret she had been prescribed HRT belatedly, and it had brought some relief of the back pain, together with the hope that things would get no worse. But nothing would straighten her spine again, or bring back the lost inches, and she remained depressed because she knew she looked older than her years – and felt it.

Loss of height is one of the obvious indications of serious bone loss for which you and your doctor should be on the look out after your menopause. You will probably know your full, adult height, when you stopped growing around the late teens. But if you're not sure of this, it can be worked out by measuring your arm span. The arms should be extended sideways and the measurement taken from mid-fingertip to mid-fingertip. This measurement is usually, though not invariably, equal to a person's full, adult height. So if your present height is deducted from your armspan measurement, this will tell you how many inches, if any, you've lost. A regular check on height could usefully become part of routine medical examinations for all women around menopause age and in the years following.

Another clue that can raise the index of suspicion about possible excessive bone loss is transparent-looking skin. This is the result of collagen loss, just as porous bone is the result of calcium loss. Many doctors, including John Studd, a leading gynaecologist who pioneered HRT in this country, insist that there is a close correlation between these two conditions.

Mr Studd told me, 'All women experience progressive loss of body collagen after the menopause which produces thin, dry skin, brittle nails, aching of muscles and bones and loss of the collagen connective tissue matrix of bone. It is this change which is the fundamental cause of osteoporosis, because the collagen "scaffolding" is lost and the bone mineral disappears, leaving bone strength greatly diminished.'

For this reason, measuring the thickness of the skin

on the top of your hand can usually provide a pointer as to whether bones are unduly thinning at the same time. It is a simple test, using calipers, that an informed GP can easily do in his surgery. A more accurate method is to use an ultrasonic measurement device.

Periodontal disease, with receding gums and loosening teeth, can sometimes be another alarm signal. An X-ray, carried out by your dentist, which shows bone loss in the jaw area, can often hint at reduced bone density elsewhere in the body.

On the whole, however, although they are sometimes still used for this purpose, ordinary X-rays don't really pick up early bone loss very well, even when applied directly to the most vulnerable osteoporotic sites, such as the hip and spine. The problem is that the hard, dense outer layer of cortical bone tends to obscure loss from the inner honeycomb-type trabecular bone, the type most affected by post-menopausal osteoporosis. It's estimated that until thirty per cent of bone mass has gone, there's no guarantee that ordinary X-rays will register the problem at all. By then, of course, the damage will have been done and it could be actual fractures or distortion of the vertebrae that show up in the pictures.

In contrast, the latest, more sophisticated, screening methods can identify thinning and porosity of bone very early, and right at the areas of most risk. By repeating the screening process after a set interval, doctors can also calculate the *rate* of bone loss – a factor already noted as vital in assessing the degree of osteoporosis risk and determining the type and extent of the counter-measures required.

Unfortunately, much of the high-tech equipment involved (such as specially modified CAT scanners) is extremely expensive and not yet available in all areas. However, increasing numbers of specialist centres around the country are now becoming variously equipped for bone density checks and referral to them should become more and more feasible in suspect cases. As awareness of the current osteoporosis crisis grows, and there is fuller recognition among doctors that modern medicine has practical ways of preventing or at least controlling the problem, screening for bone loss will become more widespread.

In the last few years, more specialized machines, collectively known as densitometers or absorptio-meters, have been developed and, being both less expensive and more precise than even modified CAT scanners, they are likely to prove powerful weapons in the battle against brittle bones and further encourage the concept of routine screening.

Before describing these new screening devices and techniques, it's relevant and interesting to look back briefly at the original method of detecting post-meno-pausal bone loss. It is a method still sometimes employed, and as a research tool it was of enormous historical importance in the HRT saga. It was studies done by this old method that provided evidence con-vincing enough to persuade British doctors that osteo-porosis in women *was* linked to oestrogen deficiency and that it *could* be prevented by oestrogen replace-ment.

Let's look back for a moment to 1972, the year that a strange story was first picked up on the Fleet Street grapevine. Rumours began to circulate that something called Hormone Replacement Therapy, which could completely eliminate menopause problems, was already in wide use in America, Europe and Japan, but was being deliberately denied to British women! It was the ever-vigilant *Telegraph* that asked me to investigate and evaluate this claim. From the initial research I did among doctors in this country, it became immediately obvious that not only HRT but the meno-pause itself was being completely neglected in Britain.

Little or no research was being done, few women had even heard of HRT, and few doctors *wanted* to hear.

This attitude did not seem too surprising when I discovered that our medical schools were still teaching young doctors that because ovarian failure inevitably happened to all women, it was natural and required no treatment! Noticeably, the same argument was *not* applied to other common degenerative changes – to declining hearing, failing sight, decaying teeth – all of which afflicted *both* sexes as part of the normal ageing process.

One way or another, it became rather difficult not to suspect that if men suffered an abrupt physical menopause, with atrophy of sex organs in early middle age, falling hormone levels, failing libido and crumbling bones, they might not have been quite so ready to write it all off as natural. An alternative, like HRT, would almost certainly have been tried, tested and widely used.

Some of the more compassionate GPs here did prescribe pain killers or tranquillizers to try and relieve severe menopause symptoms, and just a very few avant-garde doctors even went as far as prescribing oestrogen for a few weeks. This sort of cat-and-mouse treatment brought magic relief while it lasted, only to plunge the poor patient back into the old misery when the short course ended. In the main, however, women who dared to complain about menopausal problems were simply told: 'It's just your age. You must put up with it'.

The exceptions to this laissez-faire philosophy, as far as I could discover, occurred only in the private sector. There I found many top specialists displaying a very different attitude. They certainly didn't write off severe menopause symptoms as 'natural', or expect their patients to put up with them. They were well informed about HRT and understood its long-term value in protecting bones, so that they were willing to prescribe it not just for a few weeks but for five or ten years to ladies who could afford to pay.

Fortunately, for the rest of us, one of the men I met there was Sir John Peel, then the Queen's own gynaecologist, and as it turned out he felt as strongly as I did that this treatment should not remain privileged medicine but be available for *all* who needed it. It was the open support he gave me, allowing me to quote him and eventually writing the Foreword to *No Change*, that helped to give HRT the respectability it so badly needed in those early days, when the majority of our conservative medical profession was still dismissing it as some money-making American import, unproven in value and unsafe in practice.

The story of the fight to change British medical attitudes toward the menopause and HRT is explained fully in *No Change*. Each new edition has had to be updated to follow the on-running drama, the various scares, the set-backs, the triumphs and the great advances in techniques and safety developed over the last decade. It has been particularly satisfying to record the vital research, carried out here in our leading NHS menopause clinics, which succeeded in solving the outstanding problems and overcoming the fears that had worried doctors, eventually providing guidelines for safe administration that are accepted worldwide. By the early 1980s this work had taken us from the bottom of the HRT league to the top, as far as technical know-how is concerned.

To the great credit of women, the NHS clinics where this important research was carried out came into existence largely as a result of pressure these women brought to bear. Once women learned about HRT, understood its logic and recognized its benefits, their demands for treatment became overwhelming. Family doctors were besieged, but were mostly unfamiliar with

Hormone Replacement Therapy for the menopause both in theory and practice. So British medicine was forced into action and the response was perfect – a network of special clinics was set up to accept GP referrals, prescribe HRT where appropriate, and then carry out much-needed research and monitoring on growing numbers of patients.

Today, although more and more GPs prescribe HRT and have good safe methods at their disposal, both NHS and private menopause clinics still function with research still going on, as it should in all dynamic fields of medicine. An up-to-date list of clinics is detailed on page 177, as well as in *No Change*, together with the addresses of other agencies helpful in obtaining treatment.

Although I don't want to repeat the HRT story here, I do want to describe one bit of HRT research, which I found already underway in Britain in 1972. As it happens it was directly concerned with osteoporosis and destined to exert considerable influence in persuading doctors to take HRT seriously.

In the early seventies, at the Mineral Metabolism Unit at Leeds General Infirmary, I found a team of doctors under Professor Chris Nordin busy with studies which would eventually provide the proof positive that increased post-menopausal bone loss was directly linked to oestrogen deficiency and could be prevented by oestrogen replacement.

With no modern sophisticated machines to help them, the researchers had to identify and estimate the increased bone loss by painstakingly measuring any rise in levels of calcium excreted in urine. This measurement always had to be made after a twelve-hour, overnight fast to ensure that none of the calcium came from food, but all came simply from the bones of the body.

The results I saw on my several visits to Leeds were impressive and when the papers were published they certainly impressed the more open-minded doctors.[1] They clearly demonstrated a tenfold rise in levels of calcium in urine, taken from groups of women suffering early natural or surgical menopause, compared to levels from control groups of women of similar age whose ovaries were still intact and functioning. Significantly, this rise paralleled the tenfold rise in Colles' fractures of the wrist already recorded in women following the menopause.

Even more importantly, however, by replacing the oestrogen that the women in the post-menopausal group no longer produced, the Leeds work went on to show that calcium loss could be brought back to pre-menopause levels. In other words, HRT could prevent increased bone loss.

Over the years these results were to exert great influence on gynaecologists and GPs in this country. Not only were they striking in themselves, but Chris Nordin, in charge of the work, was one of the world's leading experts on calcium and bone metabolism and in great demand as a speaker at the special menopause seminars and post-graduate courses that began to proliferate as interest in HRT grew. I was lucky enough to be invited to talk at many of the same meetings and registered the enormous impact his logical and articulate contributions made, particularly backed as they were by his convincing graphs.

Unfortunately, since taking up the post of Clinical Professor at the Royal Adelaide Hospital in Australia, Professor Nordin has been lost to this country. But at least he's still continuing his work on osteoporosis and HRT, and I suspect it's no coincidence that HRT treatment rates have risen steadily 'Down Under' during the years he's been out there.

In the sixties and seventies, the Leeds team were among the first to do work that proved oestrogen replacement could prevent bone loss. Confirmation continued to come, however, from other studies carried out here, particularly from work by Drs Aitken, Lindsay and Hart.[2] In America, I had also met Dr Gilbert Gordan, who had carried out similar studies in that country with similar results.[3] It all added up to such overwhelming proof of the effectiveness of HRT in preventing post-menopausal bone loss that I knew I must fight for this treatment. And not, as I'd first thought, just to help women overcome the usual and obvious menopause problems (though that had seemed reason enough to go into battle) but more importantly to help them preserve what Chris Nordin called 'a positive calcium balance', the condition essential if bones are to stay stronger for longer.

Screening methods used today

Urine and blood tests: The urine tests just described are still used today, though far less often than in the past, because they don't provide a totally definitive test and certainly cannot quantify the *rate* of bone loss so important in assessing ultimate osteoporosis risk. Analysing bone breakdown products from urine, however, continues to be helpful in distinguishing between bone loss due to osteoporosis and that caused by other disorders.

Blood tests serve a similar purpose. Abnormal levels of calcium, phosphorus and a special enzyme (alkaline phosphatase) concerned with calcium metabolism do not indicate osteoporosis in the post-menopausal woman, but they do often provide a clue to some secondary cause of excessive bone loss, such as over-active thyroid or parathyroid glands, or the condition called osteomalacia, where bone is softened through deficiency of Vitamin D.

Single Photon Absorptiometry (SPA): I first saw this

method employed when I went to lecture at the Center for Climateric Studies at the University of Florida in 1983. Since then SPA has become widely used in America and is also available in a few specialist centres here, although it's being gradually overtaken now by better and more cost-effective techniques.

Where SPA systems exist, however, the method is still used. It's based on calculating the mineral content in the bones of the forearm (radius and ulna) by measuring how many gamma rays are absorbed. The greater the mineral content the greater the bone density and the greater the absorption of gamma rays. A computer calculates and prints the results out in graph form, the whole test taking less than ten minutes. The test is quite painless and has the great advantage of exposing the patient to less than one-hundredth of the radiation of an ordinary X-ray.

There are, however, drawbacks and limitations. Firstly, the machines are relatively expensive and, although this technique can detect bone loss as low as one per cent to three per cent (compared to thirty per cent with ordinary X-rays), its greatest accuracy is confined to the mid-point of the arm. Measurements there correlate well enough with the possible condition of the neck of femur, because the radius also consists mostly of cortical bone. But to get results which correlate well with the spine, where the vertebrae have a high trabecular bone content, it's necessary to take measurements at the lower end of the radius, where twenty-six per cent of bone is also trabecular. Unfortunately, at this mid-point such measurements are not generally as consistent and precise.

Dual Photon Absorptiometers (DPA): These more complex machines to a great extent overcome this problem but are even more expensive. They do, however, provide a practical method of measuring trabecular bone in the spine. Originally confined, because of cost, to research, they're now used (where they are available) for diagnostic and bone density assessment purposes. The principle is the same as for the Single Photon system, except that an isotope is used with two energy sources. This allows accurate measurement of bone density at deeper trabecular level. Again, radiation exposure is very low. Although the cost is higher than for Single-Photon Absorptiometry, it is less than for a CAT scan. Some DPA systems exist in Britain.

CAT scanning: Until recently, the most accurate way of measuring early bone loss was via a CAT scanner specially modified for the purpose. Most people will be familiar with this marvellous type of machine which uses a revolving X-ray source to produce pictures section by section through the body, like slices of salami. These are displayed on a screen and can also be transformed into a print-out. CAT scanners are extremely expensive and involve rather high doses of radiation. At the moment there are not enough of them (with or without the necessary modifications required to measure bone density) and it would be too expensive to use them for routine preventive checking or monitoring of treatment. It would also be unwise to expose patients without very good reason to rather high radiation levels. But CAT scanners are very valuable in suspect cases where the diagnosis is not certain.

Dual X-ray Absorptiometer (DXA): This is the latest and most hopeful development so far in bone density assessment. It uses dual energy pulsed X-rays, rather than isotopes, and these produce images of higher intensity, greater resolution and greater consistency and precision. The scan speed is also much higher so that it is more cost-effective, taking far less time than a CAT scan while giving even better results. The radiation exposure is also far lower (less than one-tenth of even a normal chest X-ray) and DXA equipment can be installed in an ordinary examination room without any need for shielding or special provision of that kind.

The standard machine achieves local spine or hip scans in only five minutes, while a special whole-body machine can measure whole-body calcium in under five minutes and carry out local spine scans in less than thirty seconds. So, for the first time, all this really makes routine screening for early osteoporosis practical and DXA facilities are proliferating across the country – at least three firms are now manufacturing this equipment and, in 1989, one reported their Hologic Bone Densitometers already installed at nineteen centres in Britain.

There is a school of thought which dismisses the concept of routine screening for osteoporosis as involving unnecessary cost. They argue that HRT is such an effective form of prevention and now so safe that, with one woman in four *known* to be at risk, it is more economic simply to give hormone replacement on a prophylactic basis to all women as they begin to lose ovarian oestrogen, rather than bother to screen out those at especially high risk.

It is a very persuasive argument and no one could be more enthusiastic about HRT, or more aware of all the other benefits it brings *in addition to* protecting our bones, than I am. All the same, it's a fact of life that some women prefer *not* to have any form of medication, even hormones that are perfectly natural to the female system, *unless* they are convinced it is absolutely necessary. Detection of high osteoporosis risk provides a compelling reason for treatment, and therefore for some women a system of accurate screening is going to be vital to any decision.

But also relevant to the decision about whether or not to be on HRT is a good understanding of how this therapy works and the choices in treatment methods available today. So, for anyone contemplating HRT now or in the future, the next chapter will outline the risks, the benefits, the few contraindications and the variety of ways HRT can now be given, with the advantages and disadvantages of these different routes of administration compared.

Chapter 5

Hormone replacement therapy

By this stage, the basic concept of HRT will be clear – it is simply a matter of making up the oestrogen deficiency that occurs once the ovaries shut down. But before looking at the different ways in which this can be done today, a little explanation is needed to discover why – whichever method of administration you and your doctor decide upon – *both* hormones must always be used if you have *not* had a hysterectomy, or, to use the medical jargon, if you have an 'intact' uterus.

It's very important to understand the reason for this, because most women, including myself, actually feel at their brightest and best on oestrogen only. It is this hormone, rather than the second female hormone, progesterone, that is responsible for the great boost to mental and physical well being associated with HRT. It is also oestrogen which eliminates flushes and other symptoms, and which is responsible for bone protection, although some studies have indicated that some synthetic progestogens can also help, and may even encourage, the laying down of new bone.[1]

Unfortunately, there is a problem in using oestrogen on its own for any length of time. After the menopause it does *not*, of course, make you fertile again but it does continue to do its old job of building up the lining of the womb ready to receive a fertilized egg – just as if ovulation *really* were still possible.

During our fertile years, in each normal cycle the ovaries produce first oestrogen and then, in the second half of the cycle, the other ovarian hormone, progesterone. This second hormone modifies and preserves the womb lining, further preparing it for the possible implantation of a fertilized egg. But if no conception takes place, the supply of progesterone is cut off and oestrogen levels also drop. It is the fall in progesterone, however, that provides the really powerful trigger that causes the build-up of womb lining to shed, together with the unfertilized egg. This is menstruation.

On HRT, after the menopause, it is equally important to ensure a similar regular and complete shedding of any womb lining that has been built up. Without this 'menstruation' – or 'withdrawal bleed' as it's more properly called at this stage of life – unwanted and unhealthy thickening of the womb lining can occur. From the start experts feared that in a few cancer-prone women this condition (hyperplasia) just *might* offer a pathway for uterine cancer.

In the early days, although such fears were only hypothetical, the men who pioneered HRT in America advised the use of *both* hormones as a logical safety measure. Oral progestogen was recommended to be taken alongside oestrogen for the last part of each cycle. This closely simulates the natural hormone pattern of the fertile years, and the withdrawal of the progestogen at the end of each monthly course would provide the same sort of powerful trigger and produce the same obligatory shedding. Where this was done, it all worked to plan and the withdrawal bleed, although very similar to menstruation, proved in most cases to be both lighter and of shorter duration.

It would have saved a lot of worry for a lot of women if the experts' advice had been heeded and this 'combined' system of HRT had been adopted from the beginning in America. Instead, because women there can often dictate to their doctors exactly what they want (in a way that we can't in the UK), very many of them opted for other systems of HRT that excluded the use of progestogen. They knew they felt better on oestrogen alone and, also, in this way they could often avoid the inconvenience of a monthly bleed. If their physicians would not agree to this, then they were prepared to just take their menopause and their cheque books elsewhere.

Presumably, because the risk involved in using oestrogen alone was then only considered theoretical, it was not sufficiently emphasized or explained. Certainly, among the women I met and talked to over there, I found that the majority were on oestrogen alone, sometimes continuously, which totally avoided a bleed, but mostly on a system of three weeks on and one week off. This was a convenient compromise. Doctors assumed (and no doubt believed) that if there was any real build-up of womb lining, then the drop in oestrogen levels during the week-off treatment would be sufficient to produce the corrective shedding.

Unfortunately, this assumption proved to be over-optimistic. In 1975, the alarm bells began to ring in America. Hypothetical risk suddenly become real risk. Retrospective studies in the US were published that indicated a small but statistically significant increase in endometrial cancer (cancer of the lining of the womb) in women on oestrogen, compared to untreated women of the same age.[2]

No change includes a very detailed account of all these studies for anyone who wants the full facts. But to summarize briefly, when gynaecologist Joe Jordan and I telephoned America and spoke to Dr Donald C. Smith of Seattle, the man who had carried out the largest study, we found that the scare had been considerably exaggerated. When we established the actual categories of cancer involved, our experts here considered that many of them did not even rank as early cancer, but only reversible 'hyperplasia'. Nevertheless, it caused something of a set-back in the acceptance of HRT among GPs in Britain, just at the time when they were showing real interest. It had even more impact in America itself, although even there the scare proved only temporary and today HRT is being widely prescribed again – though considerably more carefully this time round.

It's important to emphasize that the same prescribing mistakes were *not* made in this country. Also, luckily for me, *No Change* had from the first put across the combined therapy message. This was due to the good advice I'd had from Robert Wilson, the British-born gynaecologist who first pioneered HRT in America, and from Professor Robert Greenblatt, at whose famous HRT clinic in Augusta, Georgia, I'd spent several days, meeting patients and, with their permission, watching the great man at work. My book quoted both doctors firmly advocating the 'combined' therapy, and this was strongly reinforced by similar advice from our own Sir John Peel, who insisted that the addition of a progestogen course was the only safe way of prescribing, if over-stimulation of the womb was to be avoided.

Fortunately, even before the 1975 American scare, our NHS menopause clinics had started research to answer important, outstanding questions. With traditional thoroughness British medicine was not content to deal just in hypothetical risks and theoretical protection. It wanted the facts. To get them, three of our leading clinics carried out biopsies of the womb lining of every woman they dealt with both before and after treatment with varying regimens of HRT. In this way they were able to confirm that on oestrogen alone, even with a week off treatment in every cycle, just a few women *did* develop hyperplasia. In all cases the condition completely regressed on treatment with progestogen.[3]

Even more importantly, these British studies went

n to establish that ten to twelve days of progestogen gave optimum protection to the womb lining. As a result, regular progestogen courses of that length, taken alongside oestrogen in each cycle, became part of good prescribing. The pharmaceutical companies responded by incorporating these into their 'combined' packs, something which made HRT easier for doctors to prescribe and for patients to take. As confidence in this method grew, and the safety factor of the progestogen course was confirmed by monitoring, it was no longer found necessary to stop oestrogen intake even for a week. This proved a considerable advantage to those women whose symptoms tended to return in even that short time.

So, although we came to HRT more slowly here than in America and Europe, we came to it with more thorough research behind us so that safer practices were used from the start. Indeed, results feeding through today from on-going studies show less endometrial cancer in women on modern combined HRT than in *untreated* women of the same age.[4] Doctors are now so confident of progestogen protection that even the biennial biopsy, once thought advisable to check the condition of the womb lining, has now been abandoned.

Our clinics also demonstrated that if the reason for the progestogen course was properly explained to patients, and the safety factor understood, ninety per cent of women accepted the regular scheduled bleed as a small price to pay for the benefits HRT conferred.

It is important for women on HRT to be aware that any *unscheduled* vaginal bleeding should be reported to their doctor. For women *not* on HRT, *any* bleeding in the post-menopause must be considered abnormal, requiring investigation, as it can sometimes indicate a malignancy.

Another point worth stressing is that younger

women, who may start HRT while still occasionally menstruating, need to be aware that replacement therapy does *not* give contraceptive protection. There is often some confusion about this fact, and between HRT and the Pill.

Differences between HRT and the Pill

The confusion between HRT and the Pill arises because many women know that both are based on oestrogen and progestogen. There is a big difference, however, between the types of oestrogen involved – and the dosages. Modern contraceptive Pills are now very low dose compared to the early Pill, but HRT requires even lower doses of oestrogen, only a quarter to an eighth of that needed in the Pill. HRT is effective against menopause problems at an oestrogen level too low to inhibit ovulation, and this very low dosage allows safe *natural* oestrogens to be used. In contrast, to prevent ovulation the Pill has to employ higher dosages that require powerful *synthetic* oestrogens, and it is these that have been implicated in the slightly increased thrombosis risk associated with Pill use – particularly in older women and in women who smoke.

The other important difference between the two is that the hormones in the Pill are *added* to existing hormone levels, while those for HRT simply *replace* missing hormones.

GPs could help a great deal by explaining this contrast more fully to their patients, when discussing HRT. For younger women it would provide a useful warning that being on HRT does not exclude the need for effective birth control as a precaution against unexpected ovulation. The latest advice is to use some form of contraception for at least two years when the menopause occurs *before* the age of fifty, and for one year when it occurs *after* fifty.

For older women there would be considerable reassurance in understanding exactly *why* it is wrong to extrapolate increased thrombosis risk from the Pill on to HRT. The *British Medical Journal* made the position crystal clear when it published chapter and verse with a review of all the evidence by some of Britain's top experts in the HRT field.[5]

This concluded quite firmly that thromboembolism is not increased in women taking natural oestrogen after the menopause.[5]

How HRT can be taken

It is probably clear by now that any woman without a womb to protect can take HRT in its simplest form, just using oestrogen alone. In the context of HRT these women have the best of both worlds – the benefits of oestrogen, with the energy and sense of wellbeing it confers, without the regular interruption to this buoyancy that the progestogen phase sometimes induces and, of course, without the inconvenience of any withdrawal bleed.

For the rest of us with wombs to protect, whichever way we may choose to take our oestrogen out of various established methods described below, it's still necessary to take a progestogen for ten or twelve consecutive days in each cycle.

Oral method: Taking daily tablets of natural oestrogen by mouth remains the most common form of HRT and the method most often prescribed by GPs. It proves a very successful system for the majority of women, combining good control of dosage with the ability to stop treatment easily in the rare event of this being desired.

There's a choice of HRT products available, either with progestogen built-in, or *without* this second hormone, to cater for hysterectomized patients or to allow doctors to prescribe a progestogen of their own choice. All come in at least two strengths and, as in all good medicine, the cardinal rule is to use the lowest effective dose. But remember, the dose effective enough to relieve flushes may sometimes not be sufficient to guarantee bone protection, so check this point with your GP.

Examples of the minimum effective doses offering good bone protection are 0.625mg daily of Premarin (conjugated equine oestrogen) or 2mg daily of Pro-gynova (oestradiol valerate). Both are naturally occur-ring oestrogens.

In combined form (with the progestogen content built in) these two names change to Prempak-C and Cyclo-progynova respectively. But there are many other good brands, such as Trisequens, and a full list is detailed on pages 80–81. All you really need to confirm with your doctor is that a *natural* oestrogen is being prescribed, that the dosage is enough to prevent bone loss, and that if you have a womb to protect you are also being given a progestogen.

More and more, the state of the art in modern replacement therapy involves tailoring the treatment to the individual patient and her individual life style, with regard both to dosage and to the route of adminis-tration.

The transdermal patch: This is a relatively new system which literally involves a small transparent patch impregnated with natural oestrogen being stuck to the skin of the lower abdomen or hip. The patient does this herself and must renew it twice weekly. It is a good idea to apply the patch to a slightly different area each time, when changing it, to avoid any risk of the slight local skin irritation experienced by some women.

If this problem proves to be rather more than slight, or very persistent, then the patch is not for you.

For the last ten days of each monthly cycle, a progestogen tablet must be taken if you have not had a hysterectomy. Research is underway to find a form of progesterone that can be absorbed through the skin in the same way as the oestrogen, allowing a 'combined' patch to be produced. Latest news indicates that this may be available before too long and clinical trials are already underway.

The great advantage of the patch method is that it avoids the slight loss of oestrogen in the digestive tract that occurs with the oral method. The transdermal route means the hormone is absorbed through the skin straight into the bloodstream and this allows a lower dosage to be effective. The *disadvantage* is that the patch sometimes comes adrift, especially in hot, humid climates and very occasionally during intercourse. It is not entirely unknown for the husband or male partner to end up wearing the oestrogen by mistake, an adornment not likely to help his libido or anything else. This is however a rare occurrence and one easy to avoid once you are aware that it can happen. Happily, the patch at the right dosage has proved to be protective of bone, the minimum effective dosage for this purpose being Estraderm 50. GPs are prescribing this method to patients more and more often and it's particularly useful in the rare instances where digestive problems occur on oral HRT or where there is a raised blood pressure problem.

The subcutaneous implant: Like the patch this method bypasses the digestive tract, allowing a slow release of oestrogen for up to six months. Unlike the patch it is *not* available from most GPs, although some are now giving implants and it's a technique fairly easily acquired, as it involves only local anaesthetic and very minor surgery. A pellet of natural oestrogen (oestradiol) is inserted through a special tube (a cannula) into the layer of fatty tissue just below the skin, usually in the lower abdomen or buttocks.

The whole implant process is quite painless, takes only a few minutes, and lasts for up to six months. Progestogen, of course, must still be taken orally for the first ten or twelve days of each month by any woman who has not had a hysterectomy. So far, it has not proved possible to give this second hormone successfully in implant form. There is, however, the option of having an implant of a small amount of male hormone (testosterone), which can be simply popped down the cannula at the same time. This has very special benefit for any woman who feels the need for a boost to libido or general drive.

The advantages of the implant system are that it cuts the need for daily pilltaking, and provides a slow, steady release of oestrogen, absorbed directly into the bloodstream, so that again a lower dosage has to be used. The main disadvantage is that an implant cannot be easily removed if there is a good reason to discontinue HRT.

There have also been recent indications that some patients on oestrogen implants can develop what is called tachyphylaxis. This involves a build-up of tolerance to the original dosage. This can mean repeats being needed for symptom relief at decreasing time-intervals. Repeat implantation performed *too* soon can result in high circulating oestradiol levels, well above the normal physiological range. This problem is currently being investigated further but meanwhile, where repeat implants seem to be required prematurely, a routine check on oestradiol blood levels before re-implementation is a precaution now taken by many doctors, and as a temporary measure the patch can bridge the gap if some postponement of the next implant is thought advisable.

With testosterone implants, the only disadvantage seems to be a slight risk of triggering a somewhat stronger growth of body and facial hair in women who already tend to be hairy. I found this to affect only two out of the sixteen women I met at Dr Greenblatt's clinic in Georgia, and both of them insisted testosterone had brought such dramatic improvements to their sex lives that they would never give it up; they preferred simply to cope with the surplus hair.

Continuous combined therapy (non-sequential): All of the methods described so far are what is called 'sequential', with the progestogen course starting later than the oestrogen to produce a cyclic effect.

A new method, with a low dose of progestogen used continuously from day one alongside the oestrogen is now being tested. In this way no build-up of lining should occur, and therefore there should be no monthly bleed and no need for one. At the moment, pending further and larger scale trials, this system has to be considered experimental, but the evidence to date proves that it is equally effective in eliminating menopause symptoms and provides good protection for bones. If further work confirms this, and if this method provides the same good heart protection that the other HRT courses give, then such a system may well be more convenient, with special value to older women who come to HRT well after menstruation has ceased and who are more reluctant to face the prospect of a renewed monthly bleed. It will also help the few women who find that their usually light bleed drags on, or involves pain and uterine cramps too unpleasant to tolerate. Women I have spoken to, already being prescribed HRT on this new continuous combined system, are usually enthusiastic about it and it looks a promising further option. A few do experience 'spotting' which is not always acceptable.

Vaginal oestrogen creams: Two *natural* oestrogen creams are available in the form of Ortho-Gynest Cream and Ovestin Cream. Although these are designed primarily to relieve vaginal dryness, and are very effective for this, doctors and patients should be aware that the oestrogen is also absorbed through the vaginal mucous into the bloodstream to have *some* systematic effects, occasionally causing bleeding or spotting.

Although this also means some relief of other menopause systems, it's not generally as effective as the other methods and certainly does not guarantee protection against bone loss. No proper control of dosage is possible, as absorption rates differ considerably from woman to woman. It's possible there could also be some risk of undesirable effects on your sexual partner with this method, for during intercourse he will obviously be in close contact with the vaginal cream and its female hormone content – oestrogen is not beneficial to the male even in small doses, the way that the male hormone, testosterone, can be to women. Even when a woman only uses oestrogen vaginally, a progestogen must still be taken where there is a uterus to protect.

The chart on pages 80–81 indicates the common hormone replacement preparations used today. Consult this list for full details of generic and trade names, and their route of administration.

Contra-indications to HRT

There are relatively few contra-indications but they do include liver or gall bladder disease or a history of cancer, except for successfully treated cervical cancer. Elevated blood pressure that is well controlled is *not* a valid reason for refusing HRT, though it is one given by some doctors. Nor is the fact that a woman smokes. Smoking and *synthetic* oestrogens in the Pill are a different matter, because there is a synergistic effect, that is, they work together to increase quite disproportionately the effects each would have on its own, including, unfortunately, the thrombosis risk. Logically, there can be no similar synergistic effect with the natural oestrogens used in HRT because, as already explained, *they* do not increase the risk of thrombosis in the first place.

A contra-indication that should always be recognized, even by enthusiasts like myself, is a personal fear of HRT great enough to make a woman worried or uneasy about starting or continuing treatment. I believe well-informed GPs can usually dispel most of the unfounded fears women harbour – the confidence of the patient often depends on the confidence of the doctor. Hopefully, reading this chapter or looking at the subject in greater detail in *No Change* should also be reassuring.

One vague worry sometimes voiced by women themselves is that HRT is in some way 'against nature' or not 'natural' and that it must be wrong simply on that account. In fact it's far more likely that living so long *without* hormonal support is not natural – that women were intended to die as other animals do once their reproductive purposes have been served. In the past, that was certainly what happened to most women. Today modern hygiene, modern medicine and modern birth control have combined to extend our life expectancy to around eighty in the developed world. On an evolutionary time scale, perhaps, the life of the ovary may eventually catch up with this. The length of fertile life is already extending at the other end with puberty coming earlier. Meanwhile, if you analyse it, the whole of medicine has always in effect been 'against nature' – intervening, interfering, and defying it in order to

Hormone Replacement Preparations

Route of administration	Trade name	Generic name	Type	Comments
Oestrogens				
Oral	Harmogen	Piperazine oestrone Sulphate	Natural	
	Hormonin	Oestradiol	Natural	
	Questrin	Oestradiol	Natural	All contain oestrogen only and progestogens need to be prescribed separately for women with intact uterus.
		Oestrone		
		Oestriol		
	Premarin	Equine 17a Dihydroequilin	Natural	
	Progynova	Oestradiol valerate	Natural	
	Dienostrol	Dienoestrol	Synthetic	
Vaginal creams	Ethynyl oestradiol	Ethinyl oestradiol	Synthetic	
	Ovestin	Oestriol	Natural	
	Premarin	Equine as in oral	Natural	
	Dienostrol	Dienoestrol	Synthetic	
	Hormofemin	Dienoestrol	Synthetic	
Subcutaneous	Oestradil implants	Oestradiol	Natural	Again, oestrogen only; Progestogen needed for women with intact uterus
Transdermal	Estraderm	Oestradiol	Natural	

Oral Progestogens

Brand	Composition	Type	Notes
Microval	Levo Norgestrel	Synthetic	Progestogens suitable for use with oestrogens to prevent endometrial hyperplasia
Neogest	D/L Norgestrel	Synthetic	
Primolut N	Norethisterone	Synthetic	
Micronor	Norethisterone	Synthetic	
Noriday	Norethisterone	Synthetic	
Duphaston	Dydrogesterone	Synthetic	
Provera	Medroxyprogesterone	Synthetic	

Combined Oestrogen/Progestogen. Oral

Brand	Composition	Type	Notes
Prempak	Equine oestrone 17 Dihydroequilin and D/L Norgestrel as above	Natural	Continuous oestrogen, seven days progestogen
Prempak C	as above	Natural	Twelve days progestogen
Cycloprogynova	Oestradiol valerate D/L Norgestrel	Natural	Twenty-one days oestrogen, with progestogen last ten days; seven days no treatment
Trisequens	Oestradiol, Oestriol Norethisterone	Natural	Continuous oestrogen in various doses; ten days progestogen
Menophase	Mestranol Norethisterone	Synthetic	Continuous oestrogen; thirteen days progestogen

improve the natural quality of life, defeat the natural wastage and delay the natural end.

Risks and benefits

Cancer risks: The fact that a history of cancer is among the contra-indications makes some women fear that HRT could be directly implicated in causing cancer. This is not the case. The position is that excluding women with a history of cancer from this treatment is a precaution taken simply because oestrogen stimulates the growth of certain types of cells, including malignant ones if there should be any among them. A history of cancer inevitably involves the slight risk of secondaries already being present, and HRT accordingly might accelerate their growth.

With cancers of the reproductive organs, the hormone milieu does seem to play a role, though this is not fully understood as yet. However, the situation is clear enough in terms of endometrial cancer, with related studies confirming that combined HRT actually *reduces* the risk of this disease.[5]

Studies have found *no* association between HRT use and cervical cancer.[6] Where ovarian cancer is concerned, every case-controlled study into the Pill has found a protective effect against ovarian cancer, with a reduction in risk of about fifty per cent depending on duration of use.[7] A similar protective action is thought to apply also to HRT. This is perhaps the place to point out that while we all worry about cancer, osteoporosis actually kills more women each year than cervical, uterine and ovarian cancer combined.

The position regarding breast cancer is much more confused. Some studies show an increase of this disease in women on HRT,[8] while others contradict this with figures showing the incidence reduced by as much as one-third in women on combined HRT.[9] Quite recently, figures from on-going epidemiological studies in Oxford indicated that mortality rates from breast cancer were significantly *reduced* in women on HRT, though duration of use could prove to affect this apparent bonus.[10]

At the moment, it's not possible to draw any firm conclusions as there are so many complicating factors to take into account. For instance, many women included in published studies, especially those done in America, didn't start out on the now commonly prescribed *combined* therapy, but were originally prescribed oestrogen alone. So will the addition of progestogen prove to have a protective effect on the breast, as it does on the endometrium? Does the fact that women on HRT generally get better supervision allow breast cancers to be diagnosed more often in these groups? And does this also mean they are being detected and treated earlier? If so, is that why the mortality rate for women on HRT is lower? Cancer of the breast has a long latent period, and so it may be many years before the results start feeding through from enough women, whose entire HRT experience has been on the combined therapy, to allow such questions to be fully answered.

Meanwhile, the intensive research and studies monitoring women on treatment around the world continues, and it's a question of always keeping the *latest-known* benefits and risks in perspective. In 1989, at a medical meeting where I was speaking, Dr Kim McPherson of the Epidemiological Unit in Oxford proffered the following advice to over 400 GPs present – a turn-out that reflected the current massive interest in this whole subject. He told them: 'The advantages of HRT are so powerful and enormous that although one should not ignore any disadvantages, one should get them into balance and then let women decide for themselves.'

Deciding for yourself assumes you already know the facts or that your GP has the time and inclination to discuss fully the pros and cons of HRT with you. I'd like to think this was always the case, but if it isn't then it's up to *you* to ask the right questions if there is anything you remain unsure about. That is the only way any of us can play a proper informed role and make use of our part in the decision-making process. So, all in a good cause, let's look at benefits, risks and side-effects.

Benefits

Relief of menopause symptoms: Flushes, sweats, vaginal atrophy, palpitations, backache, headaches, lethargy and a strange sensation known as 'formication', which is rather like ants crawling under the skin, are among the better-known physical symptoms which HRT eliminates.

It is also effective against the mental symptoms often experienced at this time, including confusion, loss of confidence, poor memory and sudden onset of illogical depression in women who have never experienced this type of mood change before. Where no obvious reason for the depression exists, it is usually a direct result of oestrogen deficiency. A two-year study at King's College Hospital of menopausal women suffering from depression showed eighty per cent of them responded to HRT.[11]

Protection against osteoporosis: With the whole thrust of the book devoted to this, I won't labour the point here except to say that this protection is totally proven and accepted at all levels within the medical profession. Oestrogen implants have even proved effective against the severe type of osteoporosis induced by cortico steroid drugs.[12]

Protection against arterial and heart disease: That replacement therapy protects against arterial and heart disease has been one of the great recent discoveries, confirmed in authoritative studies from America.[13]

Of course, it was always something that was strongly suspected, but the evidence until recently has only been circumstantial. There is the fact that during our fertile years, when levels of oestrogen are highest, women are well protected against heart disease. By comparison, young men of the same age are forty times more likely than women to suffer heart problems! There is also the fact that along with losing oestrogen after the menopause, women also rapidly lose this advantage over men, with the rates for heart disease eventually levelling between the sexes.

Significantly, again, women who undergo a surgically induced early menopause or suffer a premature natural menopause also lose heart protection early, acquiring four times the risk that other women of the same age run of heart disease and strokes.[14] This clearly rules out simple ageing as the key factor in increased risk of heart disease, just as it did for osteoporosis, where the same increased risk was found to follow early menopause.

The majority of the studies revealing the reduced incidence of heart and arterial disease on HRT were based on the use of oestrogen alone. For this reason, further work is being concentrated on establishing whether the modern addition of ten or twelve days of progestogen each cycle reduces the protective effect. If so, then it will be a question of finding *which* progestogen reduces this all-important benefit *least* out of the many types available and the many new ones being developed.

Protection against endometrial cancer: This has already been covered in detail but it is important to remember it only applies to the 'combined' therapy. The reduction in risk has been estimated at fifty per cent.

Protection against pelvic atrophy: One of the very helpful jobs HRT performs is prevention of problems in the pelvic area. Unless there is enough circulating oestrogen, the vagina becomes dry and narrow, with the external skin tending to thin and be less sexually responsive. If this happens, intercourse is usually painful and sometimes impossible. Even after a lapse of time HRT can restore the health and elasticity of the vagina.

Another aspect of pelvic atrophy which HRT helps and which is rarely publicized is incontinence. Oestrogen deficiency can affect the mucous membrane of the bladder, with the resultant thinning of the sensitive bladder neck contributing to the urinary frequency and urgency with which older women so often have to contend. HRT helps to prevent this and also to maintain muscle tone in the pelvic floor.

Protection against cystitis: HRT also protects against cystitis and other urinary infections. Thinning skin tends to make the whole pelvic, vaginal and bladder area more liable to infection. By restoring healthy skin and muscle tone HRT guards against these problems.

When I met author and cystitis expert Angela Kilmartin in London she very much confirmed this. Her dedicated pioneering work for cystitis sufferers is well known, as are her books on the subject (listed at the back). She told me:

About one-third of women who suffer from cystitis first start the problem in the menopause or following a hysterectomy. Many of these women have had negligent medical care. Those who have had better and enlightened help from their GP or gynaecologist have made substantial or full recovery not only from cystitis but, of course, the other miserable symptoms as well. From the mildest oral tablet treatment through to the full-blown implant, HRT is extremely effective.

Cosmetic benefits: The benefits to your physical appearance are enormously rewarding, especially throughout the menopause when self-confidence can be low.

• Skin is as affected as bone by collagen loss. Collagen, which is part of the framework of bone, also forms a supportive network for skin. After the menopause, calcium is lost from the bone just as collagen is lost from the skin, which causes it to sag. Loss of oestrogen, as we have seen, can also result in very dry skin, with an increased tendency to wrinkling and flaking. Restoring oestrogen helps to slow down the process, and a study at a London Hospital in 1983 showed that skin quality was very much better maintained on HRT, with treated women having thicker, less-transparent skin and fewer lines.[15]

Personal testimony can be convincing and in this case it is my own. I ran into a striking example of oestrogen's benefit to ageing skin which I had not even realized. I found out about it when, after twelve years or more on treatment, I decided to tail it off. I felt my bones had had sufficient protection and I rather fancied cutting out the slight inconvenience of a monthly bleed. Within a few months I ran into intense skin irritation. It was worse on my legs and I couldn't wear nylons or slacks. Admittedly, we had not long returned from a holiday under hot sun, but in the past I'd always been able to sunbathe ardently without any problems. This time, I did notice things were different. Tanning didn't take place evenly and was preceded by tingling and reddening – not actual burning, which would have warned me, but a sort of sensitizing which for the first time in my life made contact with anything but cotton miserable. Back in England, the irritation continued, and I finally went to a dermatologist who diagnosed 'sudden and intense drying of the skin'. It was a gynaecologist friend who suggested it might all be linked to coming off oestrogen. It was. I went back on HRT and the general dryness rapidly improved, although some of the sun damage done to my skin during that time off oestrogen has proved irreversible. I certainly hadn't realized before that experience, that HRT could affect skin tolerance to the sun and to the tanning process.

● Head hair also benefits from oestrogen which increases gloss, thickness, and generally improves hair health. This can often be noticed during a healthy pregnancy, when the high oestrogen levels produce a special 'bloom' that also shows in the skin. HRT has a similar effect in many women.

● Preventing facial hair which often makes an unwelcome appearance after the menopause as oestrogen levels fall, is a very special benefit of HRT for some women. Growth occurs when the balance swings more toward the *male* hormone, something we all produce, albeit in small amounts. If the facial hair follicles, possessed by all of us from birth, are sensitive to an increased influence of this testosterone, then these follicles can be triggered. Once this has happened, it's not possible to reverse the process, although belated use of HRT may help discourage growth. Used in time, however, topping up oestrogen levels with replacement therapy prevents the problem occurring.

● Your figure will improve on HRT. One of the very obvious advantages of HRT is its ability to preserve breast shape and firmness. Without hormone replacement, breasts can become flabby after the menopause, with nipples flattening out and ceasing to be erectile. HRT prevents this, something rather well revealed in the last series of 'Howard's Way' by the shapely form of Kate O'Mara, an actress who has made no secret of being on replacement therapy.

Despite some tales of woe, HRT at the correct dosage does not cause weight gain. In fact, most women, because they feel so much better, are able to take more exercise and may even lose weight or at least retain their normal figure. At too high a level HRT can cause fluid retention and breast tenderness. The weight gain in such cases is usually only two or three pounds, and it may be worth investigating whether switching to the patch or implant, with the lower dosages involved, can overcome this problem.

Side-effects: The only unwanted side-effects of HRT are breast tenderness, and in a few women, slight feelings of nausea or abdominal bloating. These are usually transient and occur only during the first one or two cycles. If they persist, they can often be relieved by changing the type of progestogen used. Remember, the bleed is *not* a 'side-effect' but a planned and protective mechanism.

How long should you be on HRT?

From the point of view of protecting bone, the benefits of HRT are at their greatest at the time of the menopause and for the next five years. However, it is still well worth starting treatment right up to ten or fifteen years after final menstruation, when the rate of bone loss starts to go down anyway.

As we made clear earlier (see page 34), bone already lost cannot be restored (except occasionally to a very small degree) but further loss *can* be prevented. Most doctors now agree that for women who stay ten years on treatment, the onset of osteoporosis will be delayed by the same length of time. However, for women who feel well on the treatment (and most do) there is really no time limit. Women who have had a hysterectomy, of course, have no withdrawal bleeding problems, but for others contemplating staying indefinitely on HRT, it may be comforting to know that there's a tendency for this to get scantier with the passing years as the lining of the uterus becomes less responsive to hormonal influences.

At the end of an international symposium on osteoporosis held at Aalborg, Denmark, in October 1987, experts from Europe, the United States and Australia were unanimous that oestrogen was the only method of preventing this condition and that no other treatment 'stops the disease in its tracks'. They concluded that the overall effect of HRT on mortality is likely to be beneficial rather than harmful and, when given for about ten years, it will delay the onset of symptoms of osteoporosis such as fractures for the same length of time.[16]

How to get HRT

If for any reason you are consulting a gynaecologist around the time you are ready to consider HRT, then obviously it's a good idea to discuss this with him or her. In the normal way, however, your own GP is really your first port of call. He or she has the advantage of knowing your background, responsibilities and health record. With luck, these days he will be familiar with HRT in all its different forms and be prepared to discuss the pros and cons with you. This is all greatly helped, of course, if you already know something about it yourself so that you can't be fobbed off if, by any chance, you're unlucky enough to have an anti-HRT doctor. There are still some about. If you take a stand and show you know what you are talking about, it's sometimes possible to overcome old prejudices that may be vaguely persisting in the minds of some GPs, and are usually rooted in outdated fears and misconceptions.

This course of action may require quite a bit of courage, but remember, if it's successful it often paves the way for a change of heart on the part of your GP that is subsequently going to benefit many other women in their turn.

This is what happened to Mary Clarke, who was faced with a GP who insisted HRT caused cancer of the uterus. She didn't crumple up and give in, but tactfully argued that she understood the risk had been overcome by the addition of progestogen. There was a bit of mumbling and grumbling, but in the end he grudgingly agreed to a three-month trial. The results were so good that he became a complete convert; now he doesn't wait for women to ask for HRT, he positively advocates it.

More of a peril than the doctor who refuses treatment is the one who prescribes HRT carelessly and incorrectly. Joan Jenkins, Founder Coordinator of Women's Health Concern, gets some striking examples of this revealed in her vast daily postbag. When I visited her recently she showed me two letters received that very week, one from a woman who still had a womb but had been given oestrogen for years without the vital protection of progestogen, and another from someone who had undergone hysterectomy and so didn't need a progestogen, but was still being prescribed one each cycle despite all protest. It is just possible this doctor believed the progestogen had a protective effect on the breasts. If this was the case, he didn't bother to explain this.

These, I'm sure, are exceptions. Most GPs are caring and careful. But fortunately, women who do run into problems at family doctor level can find help elsewhere. If you are refused HRT by your GP, remember you have the right to a second opinion, and this can be done by referral to a gynaecologist of *your* choice privately, or under the NHS to the gynaecological department of your local hospital or any NHS menopause clinic.

If referral is refused, my own personal feeling is that you should change your doctor. But this is not always easy and at one time there was no legitimate way out of this situation except for women who could afford to go privately and talk their way in without an initial referral letter. Today, organizations like Women's Health Concern, The National Osteoporosis Society and the Amarant Trust can either steer women towards help or provide actual treatment in their own self-referral clinics.

At one time, several Family Planning Association (FPA) clinics also prescribed HRT, without any referral needed, while others acted as referral centres. Unfortunately, as from March 1990 with the takeover of contraceptive services by local Health Authorities, and the inevitable contraction of the FPA, the emphasis in their work now is mainly on advice and education. This includes advice on menopause clinics or hospitals, where HRT can be obtained in any area of the country. The address of the FPA headquarters is noted at the end of the List of Clinics, at the back of this book. One way or another, no determined woman should find herself unable to get HRT today, assuming she is found on assessment to be suitable for treatment.

As well as using HRT to prevent damaging bone loss *after* the menopause, it is important to ensure that you achieve and maintain your full potential adult bone mass in earlier years. The greater your bone density when the menopause strikes, the longer it will take, with or without benefit of HRT, for the fracture threshold to be reached. So let's look at other ways in which we can help to preserve our bones.

Chapter 6

Other strategies for preventing bone loss

Although Hormone Replacement Therapy is the only proven method of preventing post-menopausal bone loss in women, there are a number of other ways in which you can help to ensure that your potential genetically determined adult bone mass is achieved and maintained.

Compared to the very positive protection HRT gives, these additional strategies have only marginal effects on osteoporosis risk, but when you are out to defeat a stealthy and relentless enemy you need to use every advantageous ploy you can. These more general tactics apply to both sexes and are worth adopting anyway, as they not only bring a bonus for bones but some of them also for your heart.

Exercise

Apart from HRT, which applies only to women, regular weight-bearing exercise has the most direct and beneficial influence on bone density.[1] This was strikingly highlighted by the experience of the first astronauts to spend any length of time in space. On their return to earth medical checks revealed that all of them had suffered unexpectedly severe bone loss, averaging a half per cent per month during their period living in a weightless environment. Clearly, in the absence of gravity, neither the movements entailed in performing daily tasks nor the special exercises they had carried out to keep fit had exerted the stress necessary to maintain calcium balance and preserve normal bone mass.

A lesson was learned and since then, to try and overcome the problem, astronauts taking part in later missions have been set more rigorous exercise programmes using special machines and magnetic boots, designed to simulate the normal pull of gravity and create the right sort of stress on the long bones. In selecting astronauts, who early in the next century may be required to live on permanent space stations for long periods, one of the most important criteria will be that they each possess strong adult bone mass.

Even back here on earth, of course, it's been recognized for a long time that prolonged periods of bed rest or other forms of immobilization have an adverse effect on bone density, while regular exercise has a beneficial one. In one month confined to bed, as much bone is lost as in one year of normal activity with the normal ageing process at work.

Weight-bearing exercises such as walking, jogging, riding a bike or playing tennis, where stress is applied to the long bones of the body, have been shown to be of special value. Swimming is rather less effective for preventing bone loss because the support given by the water reduces the amount of stress exerted on the bones. On the other hand, it remains the activity *most* recommended where the first signs of osteoporosis are already present and a weakened skeleton needs to be exercised with special caution.

It is always difficult to think of bone being like other body tissue and reacting in a similar way, yet bones respond to exercise by growing stronger and to lack of it by growing weaker, just as muscles do. If you then consider that the heart is basically a muscle, it's logical that the physical exercise that benefits bone should also benefit the heart so that there is a double reward.

So how much exercise should you take? Going to extremes can be counter-productive for women. In efforts to keep at the top of their sport some women athletes *over* exercise to the point where oestrogen levels drop to result in a consequent loss of menstruation (amenorrhoea) *and* loss of bone. Such episodes of amenorrhoea – whether due to excess training or to other causes, such as under-eating – produce periods of bone loss in those earlier years, which means thinner bones later when the menopause strikes, thereby increasing the risk of osteoporosis.

As with most things in life, the answer with exercise is moderation, tailoring your activity to suit *your* ability, age and fitness at different stages of your life. As you grow older it's particularly important to check with your doctor first if you plan suddenly to take up vigorous sport again after not exercising regularly for several years.

Even if you restrict yourself to just walking or jogging, it's a good idea to start with some gentle exercise first, to warm up the muscles. Walking needs to be on the brisk side if it's to raise the heart rate sufficiently to exercise that, at the same time as the bones. A good plan when you first begin is to alternate brisk walking with gentle jogging for around fifteen minutes in total. You can then build up, gradually increasing the length of the jogging periods, the total length of exercise time until you're able to do twenty or thirty minutes without too much effort. Three times a week for this routine is the recommended minimum but, assuming you are basically fit, making yourself run up and down stairs instead of walking can be a good way of fitting in some extra useful exercise.

Scientific studies comparing groups of women over fifty-five who took regular exercise with others of the same age who lived sedentary lives have demonstrated that regular activity clearly does pay off in terms of stronger bones.[2] Women in their thirties and forties who play sports like tennis or badminton are well advised to keep them up. If you don't stop, you don't usually *need* to stop, even into your early seventies. And if, like me, you are competitive by nature, it's amazing how far experience and guile can compensate for some inevitable reduction in speed and mobility.

Calcium and diet

It is very important to try and get into proper perspective the role of calcium in preserving bone mass. There's been a lot of confusion about this, both in news reports and publicity campaigns. One dairy firm who advertised their 'calcium-enriched milk' as able to prevent the crippling bone disease of osteoporosis was forced to ditch this particular sales strategy when medical opinion poured public scorn on such a claim.

The truth is that adequate calcium in the diet *is* important to allow the full potential bone mass to be achieved and, until the menopause, to help maintain it. But having said that, neither calcium in the ordinary diet nor extra calcium supplements can on their own protect women against post-menopausal bone loss.

Unfortunately, this is because with age there is a definite decline in ability to absorb calcium and this probably explains the tendency for bone loss to increase to some extent in both sexes as we get older. But in women, once vital oestrogen is lacking, there is an additional decline in calcium absorption which prevents the complex processes necessary to maintain calcium balance (see Chapter Two) from being carried out.

Once missing oestrogen is replaced it may be a different matter. There is some evidence that calcium supplements or a calcium-rich diet in *addition* to HRT can be beneficial and may even allow a slightly lower dose of oestrogen to be effective in preventing bone loss.[3] Other studies have failed to show this and medical opinion is divided. Some experts in the field would certainly not concede calcium has a major role in preventing osteoporosis. However, the Consensus Conference of the European Foundation for Osteoporosis and Bone Disease (October 1987) and the Consensus Conference of the National Osteoporosis Society (October 1987) both agreed that a good calcium intake is particularly important in younger people to *establish* good peak bone mass and throughout life to *maintain* strong bones, with up to 1500 milligrams daily recommended in the post-menopausal years.

So it seems a reasonable form of double insurance if you are on HRT to make sure you are also getting sufficient calcium either from food or supplements. In deciding what this should be, experts have taken account of the fact that even normally we only absorb about ten to thirty per cent of the calcium we get either from food or from supplements. So on this reckoning, to achieve sufficient calcium actually absorbed, the recommended daily intake prior to the menopause should be at least 800 milligrams. As the hormonal changes of the menopause set in, calcium requirements increase to between 1200 and 1500 milligrams a day.

Phosphorus is another essential mineral found in every cell in our bodies, and a major component of bone along with calcium. In some way not fully understood the calcium-phosphorus ratio is involved in the degree of bone loss incurred and it's considered advisable to try and keep these two minerals more or less in balance. Because phosphorus is more readily absorbed than calcium, this means aiming at an actual intake of twice as much calcium as phosphorus.

Unfortunately, the average diet contains just the opposite balance – only half as much calcium as phosphorus. The latter is in so many of the most common foods, such as cereals, potatoes, bread, processed foods, beer, cola drinks and many additives, but most of all in meat and meat products. Cutting down on meat probably offers the single simplest way of helping to keep a good calcium-phosphorus balance in your diet and has the added advantage of helping the cardiovascular system.

Milk remains the ideal source of calcium and a glass with every meal is a good rule for children and adolescents. These days figure-conscious women and others following modern heart protection advice tend to cut down on milk because of the fat content. In both cases the answer is to go for semi-skimmed milk, for although it is low in fat, its calcium content is still good. Also, like full cream milk, it contains Vitamin D, and this too is essential for the formation of new bone. For obvious reasons cheese is another calcium-rich food and sprinkled on vegetables is just as tasty as butter and better for you.

There are some people (fewer here than in America, it seems) who have a problem in digesting milk and milk products in large quantities. This is usually due to a deficiency of the intestinal enzyme, lactase, necessary to break down the sugar (lactose) present in milk. Known as lactose deficiency or lactose intolerance, the easy answer if this condition is diagnosed is to find the level of milk you *can* take without trouble and then make up your calcium intake from other sources. For instance, a little vinegar added to water dissolves the calcium out of bones when making stock and provides as much calcium in one pint as in a quart of milk.

Apart from milk and cheese, other good sources of calcium include buttermilk, yoghurt, ice cream, broccoli, cauliflower and green beans. As a rough guide, whole foods are better than processed, and calcium absorption is helped if consumption of red meat, soft drinks (containing caffeine, such as cola, coffee and chocolate) is cut down. The following table, prepared by The National Osteoporosis Society, outlines the calcium content of a number of everyday foods.

Weight (oz)/(g)		Food	Calcium (mg)
4	112	Spinach, boiled	672
2	56	Whitebait, fried	481
2	56	Sprats	398
5	150	Yoghurt (low fat, plain or fruit)	240
⅓ pt	190ml	skimmed milk	236
3	84	cheese omelette (1 egg, 1 oz (28g) Cheddar)	235
⅓ pt	190ml	semi-skimmed milk	231
⅓ pt	190ml	silver top milk	225
2	56	sardines, canned in oil (fish only)	220
3	84	cheese and egg flan	219
1	28	Edam cheese	216
4	112	cheese and tomato pizza	212
1	28	Cheddar cheese	207
3	84	cheese sauce	201
½	14	Parmesan cheese	180
2	56	pilchards, canned in tomato sauce	168
1	28	processed cheese	168
2	56	cheese scone	140
4	112	ice cream	134
2	56	milk chocolate	123
2	56	Brazil nuts	101
2	56	Mars Bar	90
2	56	Muesli (Swiss style)	67
3	84	Suet pudding, steamed	81
1	28	Figs, dried	78
1tsp	5	dried skimmed milk (in tea or coffee)	64
½	14	Horlicks, malted milk powder	60
		1 large orange	58
4	112	baked beans	50
4	112	winter cabbage, boiled	43
1 slice	30	bread (fortified) white or wholemeal	30
⅓ pt	190	soya milk	25

Reproduced from 'Your Calcium Guide Book', with the kind permission of The National Osteoporosis Society.

If you have doubts about your natural intake of essential minerals and vitamins, there are always supplements available both on and off prescription. With your bones in mind you can get calcium combined with Vitamin D, which helps absorption, but the latter also comes in fatty fish (good again for the heart) and in butter, margarine, eggs, and liver. Sunshine, however, remains the main source of this vitamin for most of us and usually it is only older, more housebound people who suffer from any real lack.[4] Because of this, before recent health-service restrictions posed a threat to GP budgets, it was common practice for doctors to prescribe multivitamin tablets on the NHS for the over sixty-fives and these contain the daily 400 international (IU) units of Vitamin D considered necessary per day.

As a matter of some relevance to Vitamin D use, results of very new Russian and American research appear to show this vitamin playing an important role in protection against breast cancer. This is not the place for a major review but briefly, studies in both countries have shown a higher incidence of breast cancer strikingly linked to areas of low sunlight, particularly in northern lattitudes, where low ultra-violet levels means low Vitamin D levels. British work offers a rationale for this protective mechanism, as tissue cells in the breast have been found to bind very tightly together when Vitamin D is administered. Bound in this way, individual cells are hemmed in and cannot run out of control. But when Vitamin D is absent, the binding loosens, leaving the odd rogue, cancer-prone cell to grow uncontrolled. The result then can be breast cancer.

Although this is an added reason for trying to get sufficient sunlight, or making up for its lack with Vitamin D supplements, there is need for caution. Overdosing with this vitamin, instead of protecting bone, can have the opposite effect and increase bone loss. So it's never really a case of, if one tablet does you good two will do you twice as well! Even excessive calcium intake can be detrimental, adding to the risk of kidney stones in people with a history of this problem. Under 2000 milligrams daily is usually considered pretty safe but the rule with all medication, even where it is something like vitamins, considered safe enough to sell over the counter, is to stick firmly to the amount suggested by your doctor or pharmacist.

If your water contains fluoride, either naturally or added by the Water Authority, this can be as big a plus for bones as it is for teeth. Studies have shown that women who drink fluoridated water have more bone in their spines that those drinking water that doesn't contain this substance. If you live in a non-fluoride area then fluoride supplements, which come in the right, very small dosage and are cheap to buy, can be helpful in maintaining the structure of bones and teeth, being of greatest value, of course, to very young children in whom these are still forming.

The words of a song, popular long enough ago to place me firmly in the post-menopausal category, are peculiarly apt when it comes to the right strategies for preventing osteoporosis. I remember the refrain advised: '*Accentuate the positive, eliminate the negative*' and that is exactly what we need to do.

Many of the negatives to be eliminated have already been mentioned, in particular smoking and alcohol in excess: both have proved to be bone robbers. But there are a few others that can have adverse effects on bone density, including too much caffeine, which means moderating consumption of coffee, cola drinks and chocolate.

It's more surprising to find fibre, so beloved of modern nutritionists, listed among known bone robbers. In this case, however, it's such a beneficial part of our daily diet that it is not a question of cutting it out but only of allowing for the fact that fibre does limit calcium absorption. It does this partly by combining with the calcium in the intestines and partly by speeding the rate at which food passes through the digestive tract. The answer is to try not to eat the foods you rely on for your calcium alongside your fibre, and, if you take supplements, to have them an hour before a meal, two hours afterwards, or at bedtime.

Salt (sodium chloride) is essential to regulate fluid balance, maintain blood volume, transmit nerve impulses, and to other vital body processes. Unfortunately, most of us take ten or twenty times the amount we need for these purposes. The result can be raised blood pressure with increased risk of heart, vascular and kidney disease. It can also result in increased calcium loss as the amount excreted has been found to relate directly to the amount of sodium excreted. Guidelines are difficult, but one study found that on an intake of 200 milligrams of salt a day, there was no change in calcium excretion. On 2000 milligrams a day it rose significantly – 2000 milligrams is equivalent to only about one teaspoon of table salt, or just two tablespoons of tinned soup!

Personally, I find lowering salt intake extremely difficult, but stronger-minded friends insist that it can be done by gradually reducing added salt so that eventually the flavour is not really missed at all.

It goes without saying that another important negative to be avoided is drastic dieting. Most attempts to lose weight in this way result also in losing bone, because the body just takes from your skeleton the essential calcium it is not getting from reduced food. So, if you do need to go on a stringent diet for a time, it's a good idea to take calcium supplements over that period.

If all this sounds pretty daunting, remember HRT can usually prevent increased bone loss without your having to worry too much about these other peripheral precautions, though nutritional experts would consider them advisable for general health reasons.

But if HRT came into your life too late to prevent brittle bones, or maybe for good medical reasons you can't be given it, just how do you set about living with osteoporosis, assuming you are unlucky enough to be among the one-quarter of all untreated women who develop the condition? The next chapter looks at ways and means of learning to live more safely and comfortably with osteoporosis and at what medicine can do to help.

Chapter 7

Living with osteoporosis

The word 'osteoporosis' only means 'porous bones', that is, bones more porous and weaker than they *should* be for your age, sex and race. It is on that basis that your doctor or specialist could inform you that you are 'osteoporotic' or that 'you have osteoporosis', regardless of whether you have already had an actual fracture or have simply reached the sort of low-bone density level that puts you at close risk of one – what we have referred to as the 'fracture threshold'.

Either way, the first step, unless there are over-whelming medical contra-indications (of which there are few), is to get onto HRT as soon as possible. It's been stressed in earlier chapters that bone cannot be restored once lost, but recent evidence indicates that even fifteen years after the menopause, HRT can still intervene to prevent further bone loss and further height loss, and reduce the very real risk of repeated fractures. Other findings have suggested that the pro-gestogen content in the combined therapy may even stimulate the formation of new bone to some degree. Whether future studies confirm this or not, replace-ment therapy remains the recognized treatment of choice today, not only for *prevention* of osteoporosis, but for *management* where the condition is already established.

Apart from rapidly getting onto replacement ther-apy, it's impossible to lay down a single set of rules to follow for all women who may be forced to live with osteoporosis. Every case is different and so are the measures that need to be taken. Unless the condition is extremely advanced before it's diagnosed, there's no need gloomily to envisage an inevitable future of deformity and severe disablement. It *is* possible to fight osteoporosis and at least to slow it down and to limit the damage it might do otherwise.

The battle plan begins with HRT, which should halt the degenerative process, and then other strategies must be brought into play. These should include careful, correct and regular exercise, the right diet with good calcium intake and, of course, the elimination or reduction of the negative factors in your life such as smoking, salt, alcohol and other bone-robbing substances. This may involve finding substitutes, where possible, for any prescribed medications which adversely effect bone mass, or harmful over-the-counter remedies for natural, less-dangerous alternatives. For example, switching from an antacid containing aluminium to one based on magnesium, will provide relief from aluminium's bone-robbing properties. With such adjustments it can even be possible to achieve some strengthening of muscles and skeletal mass.

In working out your individual plans for managing your osteoporosis, your GP should be your chief ally. He or she will advise on what help is available, prescribe HRT, calcium supplements, and tablets for pain control, as well as referring you to the appropriate consultants if there's a question of regaining mobility or requiring specialist treatments not available through a family doctor. For example, for severe spinal osteoporosis, in addition to HRT and calcium supplements, you may be referred for physiotherapy and/or hydrotherapy – both can be helpful in relieving muscle spasm and pain, while specially designed exercises carried out in a warm water pool under supervision can also assist in restoring lost mobility.

Where HRT is inappropriate (or sometimes in addition to it) there are other somewhat more controversial drug treatments which are being used with some success in specialist centres.[1]

Calcitonin

This appears to be the most effective alternative to HRT and may prove the best substitute where strong contra-indications exist to the use of oestrogen. Calcitonin has been shown to maintain bone density, though not as effectively as replacement therapy. Unfortunately, it has the disadvantage of being both extremely expensive and – at least in the past – also somewhat inconvenient. This was because until recently it could only be given by injection. Now it is on trial in the form of a nasal spray and this may well help on both counts.

Fluoride

This is the most controversial treatment and requires strict supervision because fluoride can be extremely toxic, except at the sort of very low level found naturally in water. Nevertheless, some specialist centres have found sodium fluoride tablets beneficial in treating spinal osteoporosis, when used in conjunction with calcium.

At one time there were high hopes for this treatment because of the fact that fluoride was known to stimulate bone formation. As already mentioned, research had shown its value in water supplies and studies had confirmed that people lucky enough to be supplied with fluoridated water suffered fewer hip fractures than those drinking water lacking in this mineral.

As a treatment for severe osteoporosis, however, while fluoride increases bones density and hardness and, in particular, stimulates the formation of vital trabecular bone, problems and doubts have arisen recently because the bone produced in this way turns out to be not entirely normal or properly mineralized. It is proving to be *too* hard and *too* prone to further fracture. Also, in the doses required for effective treatment, a high incidence of gastrointestinal or rheumatic symptoms has been recorded. In addition to these disadvantages, about one-third of patients fail to respond to treatment.

Anabolic steroids

Given as tablets, or sometimes as injections, this is another therapy that, like calcitonin, works pretty well. Unlike calcitonin, however, anabolic steroids inflict definite unwanted side-effects.

These derivatives of testosterone are famous, of course, as body-building drugs for athletes, greatly increasing muscle power and endurance. At the same time they also help to build up bone. One interesting study showed that a combination of anabolic steroids and oestrogen, prescribed for post-menopausal women with osteoporosis, succeeded in actually *increasing* bone mass, while a similar group treated with placebo and another group treated just with calcium supplements alone both *lost* bone at the same rate.[2]

The problem with these male steroids at the dosage required is that they have distinct virilizing effects, including unwanted facial and body hair (not exactly popular with women). Even more importantly, they also tend to cause water retention, which in some older women may lead to heart failure. So this is a method which cannot be routinely used to treat osteoporosis, and has to be reserved for very special cases with short-term courses adopted to promote healing following crush fractures of the spine.

Self-help

Apart from doing the exercises the physiotherapist has shown you, following an appropriate diet, taking your HRT or other prescribed tablets regularly, and resolutely banishing smoking and other negative factors from your life, there are a few other things you can do, which should help to increase your comfort, protect your back, and reduce the risk of falls:

1. Check that your bed is firm and that it provides support. A plywood board under the mattress can be a cheap solution.

2. Use an upright chair or one with an adjustable back rest, which again will give support.

3. Change your position, whether sitting or lying, so that you don't stiffen up too much. If you do find yourself stiff on waking, a warm bath or heated pad can help you get going.

4. A portable cushion (fitted with a handle for carrying) can make sitting more comfortable; a small neck pillow can be invaluable if osteoporosis or arthritis is causing a painful neck.

5. Check heel height on your shoes. Lower heels are safer heels.

6. Get rid of any trailing flexes which can trip you up, even if this means extra power points. Banish all loose mats or rugs for the same reason.

7. If you have to lift, be sure to bend from the knees to save straining your back.

8. If spinal osteoporosis has resulted in any change in angle of vision, and you wear glasses, be sure to get them adjusted. Poor sight is a common cause of falls. Ensure that your glasses prescription is up to date.

9. Don't risk highly polished floors, and wipe up all spills on tiled floors.

10. Make sure lighting in your home is good, with no dark danger areas.

As well as the practical tips given above, it's worthwhile reading all you can about this condition and about all the new developments in this field. Medicine has never moved faster than it is doing today and information on new research and treatments will help to keep your spirits up. For the same reason, it often helps morale to be in touch with others coping with similar problems. There are support groups specifically for osteoporosis or for more generalized menopause problems who can help.

The National Osteoporosis Society (NOS), Women's Health Concern (WHC) or The Amarant Trust are all helpful agencies that send out regular newsletters and can advise on your nearest support group. Details of the work they do, and their addresses, are noted on pages 172–6. If you are unlucky and no suitable support group already exists in your area, perhaps *you* might consider starting one. It's extremely rewarding and not nearly as difficult as you may think. Telling your doctor and getting a note up on the surgery board, or inserting a small advertisement in the local papers tends to bring a big response. Out there somewhere are lots of others, many of them probably just as desperate as you may be for the comfort of meeting, talking and exchanging tips with other women in the same boat. Excellent information booklets, literature and regular newsletters are available from the national societies mentioned above, and special videos are available for groups, while expert talks and counselling can also sometimes be arranged.

With morale again in view, it's recognized how important it is for women to keep an interest in their appearance at a time when confidence may be especially needed. These days, there are special clothes designed to help where spinal osteoporosis produces the type of deformity that makes ordinary clothes sit badly. The National Osteoporosis Society are doing a special project on this in conjunction with the London School of Fashion and the Disabled Living Foundation. The latter give very professional advice on such matters as well as on all other problems associated with coping with physical disabilities (see page 176 for details).

Many of the case histories I've quoted are from women I don't know except through their letters, but there's one case particularly relevant to this chapter that involves a close friend of mine since school days. Jill Worrall's own first-person account is given at the back of the book (see **Women's Views and Statements**, page 130), but she was too modest to say how gifted she was at tennis, which also happens to be my own best game.

For years we were partners in doubles and rivals at singles (I remember she usually beat me), and we both played for our school, then our county and, in the heady days after the war, actually at Wimbledon.

Jill achieved this despite the fact that in her younger years she was dogged by repeated fractures and muscle problems. These were diagnosed as due to a calcium deficiency, with which she was born. 'I took every new calcium product that was produced,' Jill admitted, 'and also drank gallons of milk and ate plenty of dairy foods but I never seemed to absorb much, if any.'

Things began to improve in her teens and there was a virtually trouble-free period through her twenties and thirties, right up to the onset of ovarian decline at around forty-five. It is interesting to analyse her history, which becomes curiously significant in the light of present knowledge. It looks as though the rising oestrogen levels of puberty began to allow proper calcium absorption and eventually to provide adequate bone protection. This was then maintained and probably even further boosted by the periods of even higher oestrogen production during the years she was having her family of three children. This saw her through a successful tennis career, curtailed slightly before it need have been, so far as county tennis was concerned, when joint, bone and muscle problems started cropping up once ovarian decline and oestrogen deficiency took their toll.

'At forty-five things started catching up with me again,' Jill explained. 'It began with arthritis of the knees and then, after the menopause at fifty, came added problems in the form of generalized osteo-arthritis, back problems and pain in all my joints, particularly old injuries. The future looked black – the outlook was that I could possibly be in a wheelchair by sixty. That was when I started HRT.'

Knowing Jill so well, I've been able to see for myself the amazing difference replacement therapy brought her. She became active again, replacing tennis with golf, working tirelessly once more in her large garden, as well as coping with a big house and the demands of a growing family, including in latter years grandchildren. She has also continued to look good over the years and still does, despite having to cope with inevitable pain from skeletal damage, which once incurred usually goes on giving trouble.

Jill is sixty-six now and she remains very active, walking several miles a day with her dog, still looking after her garden and doing all her own housework. Medical management these days is somewhat against using any artificial back support but Jill does wear a light surgical corset because a disc in the area of an old sports injury has completely disintegrated, but otherwise her back is straight and quite strong.

When I saw her very recently to get permission to use her story, she added an interesting postscript. 'I do live with a considerable amount of bearable pain,' she confessed, 'but the only time it became unbearable was when my consultant suggested after ten years on HRT that I should try living without it. Within six months I had to be put on cortisone to relieve the pain and to try to keep me moving. After a further six months with things getting worse I was put back on HRT.'

Jill insists she will always stay on replacement therapy now. 'I am very little worse again now than I was ten years ago,' she said. 'Things improved enormously once I was back on treatment. I'm convinced that over the years the speed of degeneration has been considerably slowed down by HRT.'

With such fragile bones in early life, degeneration of a disc, onset of post-menopausal osteo-arthritis and a clear threat of osteoporosis in the offing, Jill was an even more obvious candidate for HRT than I was, back in 1973, when we both made the decision to go on this treatment.

But from her story, and despite all the help medicine can offer, it is clear that arthritis, osteoporosis and other intractable conditions can involve learning to live with a degree of pain. Total reliance on pain killers is rarely a good idea as the quantity needed for control can build up. But there are alternatives that can also be used; and they are perhaps worth mentioning.

Pain control

I once made a study of pain for a book I very much wanted to write on the subject. I'd completed the research, had the outline approved, the book commissioned, received the advance and begun the first chapters, when such an excellent book came out that I felt mine could never rival it. So I opted out in favour of *Conquering Pain* by Dr Sampson Lipton, who ran one of the first-ever specialist pain clinics in this country. I can wholeheartedly recommend it to anyone who has to cope with chronic pain.

Meanwhile, there are two very basic tactics worth mentioning briefly. The first is what must be termed diversionary – just trying to occupy yourself with something that takes your mind off the pain. Of course, it can't achieve miracles or blot out acute agony, but it's a successful ploy we've all seen work and no doubt used to divert children when they suffer bad falls and bumps. It can work to some extent for adults, too.

So can a sophisticated modern version of the other instinctive remedy we all use for our children and ourselves. Rubbing a place that hurts provides an alternative sensation, and this is the basis of what is called Transcutaneous Electrical Nerve Stimulation (TENS). TENS works by sending out rapid, low-voltage electrical pulses to two electrodes attached to the skin. This produces a tingling sensation, which you can control yourself to the exact degree at which it best helps to block out pain signals. This is a form of pain relief widely used now in physiotherapy departments and pain clinics, but small handy versions of TENS machines can also be bought privately for home use and cost around £70 (if you have a doctor's note which allows exemption from VAT).

It's preferable to be recommended for TENS by your doctor or physiotherapist, not only to save money in this way but because they will also ensure that you know how to use the apparatus to get the best results. It's all very simple and safe, with the individual home version incorporating a battery small enough to be carried in a pocket, and light enough if you need to use it more continuously, to be worn strapped to the body.

The scientific rationale for this type of pain relief, achieved through using a diversionary stimulant, is rather complex, but fascinating. Modern science has established the existence of a network of different nerve fibres under the skin which transmit messages to receptors in the brain. Some, called C-fibres, carry *only* pain signals and do this rather more slowly than A-fibres, which carry both pain signals and other sensations, flashing their messages more quickly. When messages from the different fibres converge for their final transmission up the spinal chord, if non-painful signals are picked up by the swifter A-fibres, they help to block the way for the purely painful ones travelling more slowly from C-fibres. It may sound complicated and it *is*, but it makes great sense as the basis for the mechanism underlying many modern methods of non-drug pain relief.

So much for what is already on offer to prevent osteoporosis or alleviate the symptoms. Now let's look at what could and should be available, even on the basis of present knowledge, and at what better prospects there may be for the future.

Chapter 8

Future hopes

Before looking at the medical developments in the pipeline for osteoporosis – and at what could be done to increase public awareness and ensure better medical provision for diagnosis, prevention and management – it's worth first briefly reporting on the progress in HRT to which we may look forward. Replacement therapy seems likely to remain the major defence for women against brittle bones and fractures in the foreseeable future.

In the past, research in this field has been concentrated mainly on the oestrogen content as the basic effective component of HRT and the target for any worries over long-term safety. The result has been production of ever better and safer oestrogens, plus development of non-oral routes to deliver the oestrogen, allowing lower, effective dosages to be used.

In the seventies, British research investigated very thoroughly the progestogen content of HRT from a purely *quantitative* viewpoint, establishing that duration rather than dosage was the vital factor in good womb protection. From these studies,[1] courses of low-dose progestogen for twelve days emerged as achieving this more fully than higher-dose courses for only seven days (previously considered adequate).

Recently, however, research attention has switched speedily to *qualitative* assessment of progestogens. This focus evolved with HRT, proven to confer protection over the long term – not only against osteoporosis, but also heart disease – it has become important to identify or develop progestogens that, if possible, do not diminish the vital cardio-vascular protection afforded by the oestrogen.

Therefore, the search is on for a progestogen that possesses good endometrial function – in other words, one that is proficient in changing the nature of the womb lining so that on withdrawal, complete shedding is triggered – but at the same time shows little, if any, negative impact on beneficial oestrogen-induced lipid changes.

If that last phrase sounds like medical gobbledegook to you, you're right. Let's try to sort it into plain English, and at the same time find out *how* the protection that oestrogen gives to the heart and arteries is thought to be achieved.

For a start, the term 'lipids' just means blood fats. The most important and the best known of these is cholesterol. By now, most of us have had it well-drummed in that too much cholesterol is a bad thing, liable to clog up arteries and increase the risk of heart attacks and strokes. So clearly, the fact that oestrogen has been shown to *reduce* total cholesterol levels must be a good thing and likely to explain, at least in part, the protective action this hormone exerts against those conditions.

But even that explanation is slightly over-simplified for there are *two* combinations of cholesterol at work. The one called Low-Density Lipoprotein (LDL), is the 'baddy' in this particular scenario, acting to *deposit* fat in the arteries. The other, High-Density Lipoprotein (HDL), is the 'goody', coming to the rescue by helping to scour the fat deposits from our arteries. Oestrogen has been found not only to *reduce* the harmful LDL fraction but to *increase* levels of beneficial HDL. In view of this fact, the ideal progestogen for HRT must be one which does not over-disturb this advantageous balance, yet still carries out its main job of protecting the womb.

Of the existing progestogens, dydrogesterone (Duphaston) would seem to fit the bill particularly well. It is being increasingly prescribed where an independent progestogen is needed, in conjunction with implants or patches. Special studies have shown dydrogesterone gives potent protection to the womb at a dosage of 10 milligrams twice daily, taken over the usual twelve-day period.[2] In addition, recent metabolic trials have indicated that, at the same dosage and over the same period, it also causes *no* reversal of the beneficial effects of oestrogen on HDL/LDL ratios.[3]

Natural progesterone itself might well have been the best choice for HRT, because it obviously doesn't affect oestrogen's protective role during our fertile life. Unfortunately, as explained earlier, it is destroyed in the digestive tract so it can't be taken orally. Nor can it be given successfully by implant as there is a high rejection rate. Natural progesterone *is* available by injection, which is both inconvenient and painful, or as a suppository which, although widely tolerated on the continent, may be considered messy and unacceptable in Britain, where an effective alternative is available. Accordingly, HRT relies on synthetic forms of progesterone, the progestogens which *can* be taken by mouth. Dydrogesterone possesses a biochemical and molecular structure closely resembling that of natural progesterone and this may explain why it complements the action of natural oestrogen so well.

Medroxyprogesterone (Provera), which also has a structure close to that of progesterone, and which, like dydrogesterone, has been around for a long time, also finds favour with many HRT experts, and norethisterone (Primolut N) is another progestogen in wide use. The most frequently prescribed progestogens in HRT remain levonorgestrel (in Cyclo-progynova) and norgestrol (in Prempak-C). But future hopes may still lie with some of the newly developed progestogens such as desogestrel, gestodene and norgestimate, which look promising but have yet to be tested over the longer term.

Coming soon

Combined patch: Already on the way and likely to be available within a year is a new transdermal patch containing progestogen as well as oestrogen, with both hormones able to be absorbed straight into the bloodstream through the skin. If current trials show this combined patch to be fully effective in all respects, *including* long-term protection of bone and heart, it could offer another welcome advance by permitting an even lower dose of progestogen to be effective.

Continuous combined therapy: Described in Chapter Five, this is already being used on a trial basis. Using continuous oestrogen and progestogen, taken daily in very small doses, has, to date, been shown to give excellent relief of the obvious menopause symptoms. What is now awaited is confirmation that it also affords the same long-term benefits for bone and heart as the sequential methods where progestogen is not given until the last ten or twelve days of each cycle.

If this proves to be the case, then it will be a popular system. It eliminates a withdrawal bleed because there is no chance for the womb lining to build and so no shedding is involved. In practice, however, some women do report a degree of spotting – not always deemed acceptable – and for the moment it must still be considered in the experimental stage.

HRT may prove even to increase bone density: Although I have been careful to claim that HRT can only *prevent* bone loss, there is growing evidence that over the years it may actually encourage bone formation. Dr Christiansen has reported that a combined preparation of oestradiol, oestriol, and the progestogen, norethisterone, given for three years, resulted in an increase in bone density of three per cent.[4] Another study from Dr Lindsay and his team, using a different oestrogen, showed an increase of between two per cent and four per cent, if treatment was started within three years of the menopause.[5] In 1988 the *BMJ* reported an increase in vertebral bone density of 6.4 per cent – achieved in just one year's treatment with continuous oestradiol and norethisterone – providing it was started within two years of the menopause.[6]

As this book goes to press, John Studd and a team of co-workers have just reported an increase in bone density of 8.3 per cent in the spine and 2.8 per cent in the hip – again, after only one year and treating patients within two years of ovarian failure (in this case using implants of oestradiol and testosterone[7]). From these results, there seems to be real hope that early use of HRT in some cases of established osteoporosis may be able to *restore* bone to at least some degree.

Calcitonin by nasal spray: Treatments other than HRT to prevent or treat osteoporosis are also still largely experimental and subject to further research. Those currently available were discussed earlier, and of these perhaps most hope rests on calcitonin. This is already used for patients where strong contra-indications to oestrogen exist, and if it could be made less expensive it would be used more widely. Trials delivering it via a nasal spray instead of by injection are under way. If this easier route of administration proves successful, with good dosage control, it will help considerably in terms of both convenience and expense. Much may then follow because once a drug has proved effective, reasonably safe, and convenient to prescribe, demand and usage inevitably increase, and the price drops. The extra experience gained from this and the greater opportunities offered for further research and studies usually result in improvements and refinements. There is a good chance this will happen with calcitonin.

Etidronate: This drug belongs to the 'bisphosphonate', or 'diphosphonate', as they are sometimes called, and promises an entirely new approach to possible prevention and control of bone loss. These substances are taken up and bond to the bone surface. Once there, they don't affect the work of the *bone-building cells* (the osteoblasts), but seem to have a paralysing effect on the *demolition* cells (the osteoclasts), reducing their ability to break down bone. There is obviously great potential in this, and the first successful trial results were published in May 1990, on cyclic use of etidronate disodium, to treat established osteoporosis. Dr T. Storm and a group of Danish researchers used the drug in double-blind placebo controlled trials involving sixty-six patients, all suffering from spinal osteoporosis and having had at least one, but not more than four, fractures. An oral dose of 400 milligrams was given daily for two consecutive weeks in every three months. To ensure adequate calcium intake, each patient also received 500 milligrams of calcium supplement every day, throughout the whole three year period of the trial, plus a multi-vitamin containing Vitamin D to aid calcium absorption.

The results showed a significant increase in vertebral bone mineral content. After only one year of treatment, there was also a marked and sustained reduction in the rate of new vertebral fractures. In addition, spinal deformity and height loss became stabilized. Most importantly, the new bone formed proved to be normal. In trials with continuous etidronate, this had not been the case.[4]

Another important study published in the *New England Journal of Medicine* in July 1990 reported research at Emory University School of Medicine in Atlanta, showing etidronate reducing new vertebral fractures by fifty per cent in women treated with the active drug, compared to a group treated with placebo. Results were even more striking in patients with very severe osteoporosis, where treatment reduced further vertebral fractures by sixty-six per cent.

Quite rightly, these results achieved on a cyclic-etidronate regimen were hailed as a breakthrough, bringing new hope for millions of osteoporosis sufferers. In the case of the two million sufferers in Britain, however, that hope is likely to be somewhat deferred. Although etidronate disodium *is* marketed here under the name Didronel, the product licence only covers its use for Paget's disease of the bone and for malignant hypercalcaemia. Before the Committee on Safety of Medicines is likely to consider an application to extend the indications to cover osteoporosis, more successful study results will be needed. It is estimated this may take at least two years.

If and when Didronel does become available for osteoporosis, its main use is likely to concern management of established disease, though it should also offer a useful method of prevention in men at risk because of long corticosteroid treatment, or as an alternative to HRT for those women for whom that treatment is contra-indicated.

For the vast majority of women, however, certainly at the preventative level, HRT is likely to remain the treatment of choice. It is physiologically more natural than any alien drug and carries with it many other benefits for women. It is also simpler to administer than etidronate, which is rather poorly absorbed orally, needing to be taken on an empty stomach with fasting continuing for another two hours to ensure adequate absorption. Such problems diminish to mere inconveniences, however, when a drug is found that actually reverses established osteoporosis, once thought impossible. For that purpose, etidronate may emerge as top choice.

A simple biochemical test to identify women at risk: A team of Danish scientists, headed by Dr C. Christiansen, have developed a biochemical test that can identify seventy-nine per cent of fast bone losers and seventy-eight per cent of slow bone losers, using just one blood sample and one urine sample, plus measurement of height and weight.

This offers great hope for the future, and recent refinement has made it more accurate. Even as it stands, if the same success rate can be reproduced by other workers (and so far it has not been), it would still mean that the majority of post-menopausal women at risk of osteoporosis could be identified at a reasonable cost. Such a relatively simple test would certainly be less expensive and more convenient than having to refer patients for bone scans to measure bone mineral content (BMC). With this method, to deduce the *rate* of bone loss, at least two scans have to be taken six months apart. While this type of scan allows virtually one hundred per cent of fast bone losers to be picked up, the biochemical system at the moment only detects seventy-nine per cent, but has the advantage of being able to do this much *earlier* in the post-menopausal period, *before* the BMC has fallen substantially. In other words, it can *predict* the problem in advance[8]. It's not yet being used routinely in the UK, but is already the subject of research and trials.

The boron effect: The effect of boron on calcium levels is currently being investigated. Scientists in North Dakota recently linked low levels of boron (a rare element found in tiny amounts in fruit and vegetables) with loss of calcium from the body. Its action has been described as that of a 'chemical watchdog', guarding calcium supplies in the body, by slowing down oestrogen loss.

In this country, the 'boron effect' is also being investigated at the Rowett Research Institute in Aberdeen, but results so far are inconclusive. Meanwhile, eating plenty of fresh fruit and vegetables each day ensures an adequate intake of some three milligrams of boron daily and may provide another form of dietary protection.

Funding for the future

With the cost to the government of dealing with osteoporosis estimated to be £800 million for 1990, it would seem economic for any promising research to be funded *and* for better provision to be made without delay both for preventing osteoporosis and for treating the established disease. The Royal College of Physicians, in their report published in 1989, make no secret of the dangerous lack of facilities for dealing with hip fractures in many hospitals, or of the need for far wider usage of HRT to prevent the problem.

In this field of medicine, as in others, it seems likely that most of the future research required will have to rely on money from the pharmaceutical industry. It is not always realized just how dependent research in this country is on the drug companies. *Sixty-eight per cent of all medical research is funded by them, with only twenty per cent coming from government sources and twelve per cent from charities.*

Without this financial investment from the drug companies, we would lack a large proportion of the medicines and vaccines which today save so many lives; for example, the vaccine that has already eradicated smallpox, and the vaccine that *could* do the same for measles – *if* the UK could only achieve the same level of take up as America, where this undere.timated and dangerous disease is now virtually unknown. Drugs resulting from pharmaceutical research have won the war against tuberculosis, leprosy, typhoid and cholera, at the same time providing a wide choice of excellent treatments for high blood pressure and ulcers which can kill, and for asthma, epilepsy and diabetes which can destroy the quality of life.

Continued funding from drug companies *and* increased funding from government sources is needed now, not just to beat osteoporosis, important as that may be, but to improve the anti-cancer treatments that are beginning to have real impact on this disease.

If this seems a slight diversion, it's one I feel worth taking, in an age when the pharmaceutical industry seems to have become the favourite whipping boy for the media. *Of course* there's a profit motive in what they do, as in all viable business practices, but while food stores are free of the charge of making profit from the hungry, drug companies are pilloried by politicians and Press for making profit from the ill – despite the fact that these profits are subject to close government control, as are their permitted advertising budgets.

My own appreciation of the value of drug company input to medicine came from the setting up of the NHS menopause clinics in the seventies. None of these would have got off the ground without financial backing from the drug companies and the result would have been dangerous delay in research that was to prove vital for the safe administration of HRT. Ironically, twenty years on, in February 1990, in the face of the evidence that HRT reduces the risk of brittle bones and cardio-vascular disease, the health minister, Virginia Bottomley, has just announced a government grant of £120,000 for research into HRT. Should we say 'too little too late', or more charitably, 'better late than never'?

In the meantime, while the pharmaceutical industry was obviously looking to HRT to make money, it was rightly looking first for maximum safety for patients as it must always do. Few powerful drugs are completely without risk and, while we seem to accept risks in surgery, we don't in our medicines. In fact, years of expensive trials precede any drug being passed by the Committee on the Safety of Medicines and, even after that, work goes on as wider experience is gained and rare side-effects are reported. This kind of research, carried out at drug company expense, can often come up with anything but welcome findings from their point of view, involving them sometimes in costly changes of formulation, as it did with HRT when the importance of twelve days of progestogen rather than seven days was established.

Almost all post-graduate meetings, designed to keep doctors updated on treatments and research, are also financially supported by drug companies. While under-funded medical schools and hospitals can provide the venues, there is no way they can find the money for fees and expenses to bring expert lecturers long distances, or provide the essentials for a full-day conference, such as coffee on arrival and some sort of buffet lunch to keep body and soul together, and brains alert.

These meetings in different fields of medicine are vital if GPs are to keep up with fast-moving modern medicine – and if valuable experience and information are to be exchanged between doctors and disciplines. They provide an opportunity not just for education but for discussion on prescribing problems, side-effects, contra-indications, patient compliance and alternative treatments. Throughout it all, the drug company involved tends to keep an extremely low profile; its particular drug may not get a mention or, if it does, it is as likely to be the subject of criticism as it is of acclaim. It's no holds barred both in the talks and discussion periods.

It's no holds barred either where the Royal College of Physicians is concerned. In their recent report on prevention and management of hip fractures, they state bluntly:

Hip-fracture patients, almost all elderly and many frail, are in danger of receiving a second-class pre-operative service. In a recent survey of 100 consecutive unselected hip-fracture patients admitted to a London hospital, sixty-six developed pressure sores. Patients lay in the accident and emergency department for up to twelve and a half hours (seventy per cent between two and six hours). Casualty trolleys in routine use were hard.

The report goes on to comment on the length of time spent waiting for operation. The same London survey had shown forty-eight per cent of patients waiting *two or three days after* admission to get to theatre, and patients prepared for surgery, waiting on the ward for transfer to theatre, lying starved and sedated for up to fourteen hours! Only one-third reached theatre in less than two hours after preparation and then, although age and injury meant these patients required the highest degree of clinical skill, they were often for logistic reasons anaesthetized and operated upon by less-experienced staff, often at night.

The report pointed out that unless special care is taken, pressure sores can begin to develop at the initial admission and 'trolley' stage. It recommended that immediately on arrival in the casualty department, patients with suspected hip fracture should be put on a soft surface (hydrophilic gel cushion or sheepskin for example) with protection for sacrum and heels. Urgent attention should be given to pain relief and to keeping the patient comfortably warm. It further recommended that, unless their medical condition precluded it, patients should be operated upon within twenty-four hours of admission and that regular daytime lists for the treatment of hip fractures should be established, to allow for careful planning and timing of pre-operative preparation and transfer to theatre, and for more experienced orthopaedic and anaesthetic staff to be available.

Considerations of post-operative care and rehabilitation also involved a long list of recommendations, and it is clear that there is considerable need for improvement there too, if the rates for premature deaths and permanent disabilities following osteoporotic fractures are to be reduced.

Present shortcomings are largely due to under-funding and resultant under-staffing, rather than to deliberate neglect. The gross deficiencies the present osteoporosis crisis is revealing are all problems that must ultimately be solved by government, the Health Service and the Social Services; greater public awareness of what is going on (or not going on as the case may be) could help bring pressure to bear for urgent improvements to be made. Teresa Gorman, the MP for Billericay, and a strong advocate of HRT, believes that women's groups could do a great deal in this respect and it's good to see that the National Federation of Women's Institutes have maintained their reputation for anticipating and tackling topical issues with a resolution passed at their 1989 annual general meeting 'to increase awareness of osteoporosis, to improve the education of women of all ages concerning the disease; and to urge HM Government to improve the advice and treatment for those most at risk. The notes published with their agenda included excellent background information, and questions discussed included how health authorities could overcome the problem of the cost of bone scanners, and whether the government should spend money on a national education campaign.

Meanwhile, as suggested in Dr Christina Kennaway's letter (printed in full on pages 150–51), education has an important role to play in the battle against osteoporosis and ideally should be started young. One hopes this education will begin at home, but while some enlightened parents will take the trouble to emphasize the importance of healthy eating, ensure regular milk and calcium-rich drinks, explain the importance of calcium to healthy bones, try to cut back on bone-robbing cola drinks and encourage exercise, in reality this is an ideal others will have neither the will nor the way to achieve. Dr Kennaway's concept, therefore, of teaching the principle of caring for our bones from nursery school onwards would seem a good one. There are encouraging signs that health care is being taught at least at infant and junior level in many education areas.

Talking to heads of primary schools, I gather it is dealt with either as part of special project work or on a somewhat ad-hoc basis, through occasional talks from visiting dietitians and nurses. Much emphasis is placed quite rightly on the care of teeth, and it would seem simple and logical to extend this to the care of bones. I suspect children would love the exercise angle and relish and remember the example of bold astronauts who have to do special exercises to counter the excessive bone loss that occurs in Outer Space. And as a practical contribution to this education, and the whole drive toward a nation with healthier bones, surely this would be the time to bring back school milk. As well as its valuable contribution to healthy bones, for some children it offers the first nourishing 'food' of the day.

All of the doctors to whom I've spoken in researching this book have made a point of emphasizing the importance of exercise at all stages of life. Dr Tom Smith, a specialist in pharmaceutical medicine who is a firm supporter of HRT, nevertheless argues strongly for the importance of exercise for women. 'Only by exercising the long bones vigorously,' he insists, 'can women build up a good "calcium bank" to see them through the calcium-losing years ahead. Women need to be physically active before and after the menopause.'

So, at least some of the things that help to protect bone are matters of simple individual responsibility and choice. No one can *make* you exercise or eat the right food but, equally, no one can really stop you. In these matters the choice is yours.

It was with those final four words that I optimistically ended the introduction to the first edition of *No Change*, back in 1975. In the event, it was to be fifteen years before the choice regarding HRT was available for *all* women.

But in 1990, as I write this book, the benefits of HRT have proved so overwhelming, particularly in regard to prevention of osteoporosis, that I believe today the choice really *is* yours. Unless there are strong contra-indications, no woman who opts for HRT should be refused. No woman who wants to protect her bones in this way should be deterred. Doctors who fail to prevent a 'preventable' disease are failing their patients and their duty.

Appendix 1

Women's views and statements

'I was born with a calcium deficiency and although throughout my childhood and teenage years I took every new calcium product that was produced, drank gallons of milk and ate plenty of dairy foods, I never seemed to absorb much, if any. Consequently I incurred many fractures and had continuous muscle problems as I was very sports-orientated. In my twenties and thirties I did seem to be stronger and it was a relatively good period of my life. But at forty-five things starting catching up with me again in the form of arthritis of the knees. Before fifty, and with the added menopausal effect, I had generalized osteo-arthritis, back problems etc. and pain in all my joints, particularly around old injuries. The future looked black. The outlook was that I could possibly be in a wheelchair by sixty. It was then I started on HRT.

I am now 66 and am still very active, walking several miles a day with the dog, gardening and doing all my own housework. My back is supported by a surgical corset because one disc has completely disintegrated as the result of an earlier injury, but it is otherwise straight and quite strong.

I do have a considerable amount of bearable pain. The only time it became *un*bearable was when my consultant suggested after ten years on HRT that I should try living without it. In six months I was forced to go on cortisone to get any relief and keep moving. After a further six months I was put back on HRT and there was great improvement again within weeks. I am very little worse now than I was ten years ago. I am convinced that the speed of degeneration has been, and still is, being considerably slowed down by HRT and I shall always continue to take it.'

Jill Worrall, Sutton Coldfield

'I am forty-nine and have been a widow for seven years. My indecision and foreboding for the future increased over the seven years rather than receding. I made many bad decisions. To this, in the last twelve months, were added severe joint pains, dizziness, crying bouts, sleeplessness, tiredness and formication.

After three months of Prempak I am restored to the energetic, decisive, sensible, painfree woman I used to be. I didn't have to persuade my doctor – *she* suggested HRT to me. Because I was still menstruating (albeit irregularly) I had assumed I didn't need it. I suppose living alone and without a family to notice how affected you are, these menopause symptoms just creep up.

I am a councillor representing an area of high unemployment and with one of the highest death rates in this country. If the over-worked, over-stressed women I represent don't get HRT at source – i.e., the GP – they are too tired, too poor and too "menopausal" to seek it elsewhere. For years contraception was the monopoly of the middle class – I intend to do what I can to make sure this doesn't happen to HRT.

To admit to any experience of hormonal disturbance is still considered a sign of weakness by many men and some women. For that reason I must remain anonymous.

A Metropolitan Area District Councillor

'When my husband presented me with an updated 1988 version of *No Change* in a Coventry bookshop on Saturday, I decided I must write to you again and tell you once more how grateful I've been for your wonderful response to the letter my husband, Vincent, wrote to you twelve years ago when, after removal of both ovaries, I suffered such severe depression that I spent six months in a psychiatric hospital. It was all useless and it was when they said they could do no more that Vincent took the initiative of writing to you.

Since going on Hormone Replacement Therapy, as you suggested, I feel I have gone from strength to strength. As I mentioned in an earlier letter, we went on to adopt three children and have led a normal, happy married life ever since.

I continue to take two tablets daily, each 0.625 milligrams. After we moved to Leicestershire last March my "new" GP did suggest that I should halve the dosage. I did this but after six weeks I had definite joint and muscle pains, with pins and needles in my arms, severe headaches (hitherto practically unknown) and a feeling of lethargy.

As my blood pressure has always remained normal, I have reverted to the old dose of two tablets daily and the muscle pain is now negligible and I feel fine.

I am now sixty-one and can truly say I feel happier and healthier than I did when I began teaching at twenty. At fifty-nine I was asked to accept responsibility for an unruly class of thirty-three children and I was able to rise to the challenge for two years until we moved to this area. Since then I have done continuous supply teaching and, this week, have been offered a teaching post for the next two terms.

Your original copy of *No Change* had to be replaced because it is still "on loan" to a person who is loath to return it. I don't blame her and I'm happy for her to have it.'

Joan Bates, a vicar's wife, Hinckley, Leicestershire

'I feel it is so iniquitous that women have often to fight

their way through the hostility of GPs to get HRT that I decided to come out publicly with my own experience. I'd seen how much my American friends benefited from this replacement therapy, and I went to the menopause clinic at King's College Hospital and got the treatment there.

That was nine years ago. I started with oral treatment and went on to implants. The results have been outstanding. The aches and pains I had been suffering in my wrists went and my old energy came back. Now I can keep going from seven a.m. one morning to one or two a.m. the next, if the job demands.

I also know that HRT is preventing the wretched bone loss that occurs after the menopause. Once gone it's never recoverable and I believe helping to prevent osteoporosis alone makes HRT worthwhile.

The implant method also improves libido and if that means that a previously happy marriage stays happy, then that's another jolly good reason in its favour.'

Teresa Gorman, MP

'My interest in HRT began in the 1960s when I was approaching my forties. At that time I was working in the BBC, and one of the women heads of service, who was vital, attractive and well past her fifties, told me she was on injections to replace lost oestrogens etc. My mother, only a few years older, had already started to break her wrist bones and became a classic osteoporosis victim. She would have benefited from HRT which could have halted this ghastly disease, but her group of GPs in a wealthy Surrey area refused to prescribe it for her. They seemed to remain uninterested in endocrinology (study of hormones) and appeared to know nothing about the vast amount of research that had already established HRT as being safe and effective when properly prescribed. Already the HRT tablets, based on natural oestrogen, had become available

on NHS prescription and combined oestrogen/proge-
stogen formulations were being given to women with
intact wombs.

In spite of my research on the subject, and my efforts
to talk to these doctors, they did nothing positive to
help my poor mother who was merely given some kind
of tranquillizers. She was quite unable to insist on
seeing a specialist and lived for another ten years with
more painful fractures and other traditional women's
health hazards.

Today – thirty years on – this same situation still
persists for countless women whose doctors misinform
them and only prescribe extra calcium or, worse still,
tranquillizers.

Needless to say, at the right time I sought medical
advice for myself and was prescribed HRT. I have
continued to thrive on it with no signs of osteoporosis,
despite the family predisposition. I started to set up
the registered charity, now Women's Health Concern
(WHC), in 1972 to try and help women in all social
classes to get authentic information about gynaecological conditions and, in particular, the menopause and
the proper use of HRT.

Dr Gerald Sawyer, one of Britain's leading consultant endocrinologists, heads our Medical Advisory
Board and a team of medical and scientific experts give
their time to fulfil our aim of improving the care of
women's health. Many hundreds of thousands of
women have written and telephoned WHC and in 1988
we answered more than 70,000 enquirers who sought
personal advice for their problems. Of these, eighty-
five per cent related to the menopause, osteoporosis
and the proper use of HRT.

But, although HRT prescribing has gone up fourfold
over the last ten years, there are still millions of women
who continue to suffer from *treatable* menopause symptoms and *preventable* health hazards such as osteo-

porosis. An important and expanding part of our work at WHC lies in medical symposia for GPs and special one-week courses for nurses wishing to become counsellors in their own districts. Hopefully this will help to improve the situation.'

Joan Jenkins, Founder Coordinator, Women's Health Concern

'I am fifty-seven and had suffered from backache for several years before last December, when I finally sustained a vertebral fracture. In the next five months I had four other similar fractures one after another. As soon as I recovered from one, I went down with another. I was virtually an invalid and for a time felt totally helpless and dependent. After osteoporosis was firmly diagnosed, I spent four weeks at the Royal National Hospital for Rheumatic Diseases, where I was put on HRT and given exercises regularly – three times a day.

I have had to be on sick leave from my secretarial job for ten months, but now plan to return part-time. I still find it difficult to bend and do simple things such as get out of bed or wash and dress, and have to be very careful not to knock myself as my bones are very brittle and will still break easily. Because of my spine crumbling so badly I have lost five inches off my height. Osteoporosis has affected every aspect of my life and it could have been so different if I had known about HRT in time to prevent it.'

Jo Lye, Batheaston

'Thank heavens I found your book! The last eighteen months had been hell with night sweats so that I couldn't sleep, palpitations, painful muscles and a crawling under the skin. At times I felt faint, dizzy and almost disembodied with ears ringing and awful headaches. The storms of weeping were quite dramatic and my depression really bad. I looked terrible. Intercourse was painful and I was just lucky to have a fantastic husband who put up with me.

I started the change five days after my fortieth birthday, nearly two years ago. My mother had started hers at thirty-nine and now has very brittle bones. She fell recently and broke her arm and shoulder and cracked her ribs. Her menopause was as terrible as mine but in those days nothing could be done.

After reading *No Change* I began a long battle to get HRT. There are six doctors in the practice, five men and one woman. I was told to pull myself together, that I was too young for the change and that HRT was not any use as it was all natural and I must put up with it.

I finally told the woman doctor that if I couldn't have a trial course of HRT I was going to go privately. It was only then that she agreed to it and even told me she had lots of ladies on the therapy and recommended it! How hypocritical of her. Still, I achieved my objective, so I don't really care.

I am now on my second month using the patch. The difference is unbelievable. I look good again. I sleep all night. All I've got left of my misery is the odd headache and some breast soreness. I am hoping that after the three-month trial period is up it will all have faded to a nasty memory.

Your book really has helped so much. Thank you for writing it.'

Mrs C. S. Roberts, South Humberside

'I am seventy-six now and had my first fracture of the knee at the age of seventy-one. Since then, I have suffered a fractured sternum, which has made the whole rib area very tender.

I don't remember at what age I had the menopause and, of course, I knew nothing about bone loss or HRT to prevent it. My GP is sympathetic and helpful but feels it is too late now for HRT to be effective. I attend the orthopaedic clinic at the local hospital, and some injections given me there recently have been helpful in alleviating the pain, but how I wish I had known about HRT in time to prevent all this.'

Mrs Bosher, Mumbles

'I am only sixty-five and because my spinal osteoporosis was not diagnosed early enough I have already reached the state where I have had to give up my home and go into sheltered housing. Thanks to Help the Aged, a flat was found in a residential home, where my husband can be with me and where there is an SRN on duty all the time. We are both grateful for this but it's not like your own home and it needn't have happened if my problem had been picked up in good time.

Because of rheumatoid arthritis I had to be put on steroid drugs at only forty-two. I also finished menstruating at only forty-seven and neither my GP nor the rheumatologist I was then under took any measures to counter the bone loss both these conditions are known to cause. Of course, at that time I didn't understand myself and, although I complained of very acute low back pain and on one occasion of extreme, agonizing pain when I coughed, it was all written off as nothing to worry about – just part of my arthritic state.

I only began to suspect something else seriously wrong when I read an article in the magazine produced by *Arthritis Care*. I was sure then that there was more to it than rheumatoid arthritis and I began the long fight with my GP to get a second referral to the Royal National Hospital at Bath, where I had been advised to go. In the end, a referral letter was grudgingly given but my GP refused to arrange any transport or give any help in that way, as he considered it all unnecessary.

In fact, the investigation revealed severe spinal

osteoporosis with two vertebral fractures already, just two inches from the base of the spine – no wonder I was in such pain.

I was treated as an in-patient for some time and still go in for regular checks and management of the condition. I was put on HRT, plus calcium and fluoride tablets and shown special exercises I have to do regularly, to try and help me keep my head up. My back is already so very bent and my ribs so pushed forward that clothes are difficult and tops like blouses and sweaters will not sit properly.

I am so grateful to the Royal National at Bath and to the National Osteoporosis Society, who do so much for people like me, that I overcame my fear and have appeared for them on TV programmes as a warning to other women. I don't want any of them to suffer as I have done when more awareness by them and their doctors could prevent it.

Sixty-five is too young to feel so old.'

Lilian Lolley, Bristol

The following are statements and views from well-known women using HRT, taken by permission of The Amarant Trust from their audio cassette.

'I had hot flushes, night sweats and found it difficult to get to sleep. I was very weepy all the time, and this made it very difficult for me to work and lead a normal life. I was one of the lucky ones regarding HRT, because my doctor said "Try these" and explained what they were. Within a couple of weeks I was fine. The weepiness took a bit longer. I must stress I wanted to *feel* better – I didn't take it because my doctor said you are going to *look better*.'

Jill Gascoine, fifty-two-year-old star of 'The Gentle Touch'

'HRT was something I'd heard about for a long time because I've always had a lot of trouble, gynaecologically speaking. It was something I knew I would probably eventually want but it didn't seem to be necessary until one's late forties. I had a sympathetic gynaecologist, so at the right time there was no problem. I've made no secret of it because I was asked outright at a press conference whether I was on HRT and had to make a snap decision as to whether to say yes or no. I thought to lie about it is cheating, somehow, and I thought I might give other women confidence if they knew I was taking it.'

Kate O'Mara, fifty-year-old actress

'Before I went on HRT, I felt very sorry for myself all the time. I had all the symptoms my readers write to me about, and that middle-aged women suffer from – hot flushes, sweats, tossing and turning all night, irritability – I was hell to live with. First I was on tablets, but they affected my digestion so I was pretty desperate. But then the patch came along and brought instant relief. Mondays and Fridays are "patch" days. I can now perform as a busy, active journalist should – I work full-time and I'm quite certain that if it wasn't for the patches I'd be like so many other unfortunate women sitting at home having hot flushes and quarrelling with the old man.'

Marjory Proops, famous columnist and agony aunt

'I'm sixty-eight and still on HRT. I take the tablets and have them every night and they are so easy and convenient. It's so simple and while I've been taking them I've never had any trouble at all. I was already fifty-seven and convinced I was going to have no bother, because I'd asked my mother about that, and she had said: "I can't tell you anything at all because I never had time for it". I was proving, however, that it wasn't all in the mind and there *was* a physical change as well. On the stage I was suddenly perspiring heavily and at night I was waking up and lying in a bath of perspiration and having what I call sort of Victorian vapours, having to hang on to the furniture now and again.

In the very early days, long before more research had been done, my doctor did say there was a very slight risk of cancer of the womb, if one was on for too long. So I thought, well all right, I'll give up because I must be all right by now. But I had to go back to HRT and she assured me by then that all the doctors had been informed that there was no worry at all. I have such a busy life, and I really don't want to stop. And I certainly won't stop because I understand it will protect me against the long-term effects of oestrogen deficiency.

It's a shame that doctors often say no one ever died as a consequence of the menopause because that is, I suspect, one of the most ignorant statements ever made, when you consider the mortality from osteoporosis, arterial disease and heart attacks.'

Dinah Sheridan, the glamorous mother, in BBC TV's 'Don't Wait Up'

'My mother, when she was ninety-six, fractured her leg and her doctor then gave her HRT. I caught my toe in a carpet in Lisbon, in a supermarket, and hit my nose and all my jewellery fell off, but I didn't break anything. I was told it was entirely due to HRT treatment. Old people's bones break like biscuits. HRT keeps the juice in them. People *do* look younger. My daughter, Countess Spencer, is sixty this year, and she looks thirty, runs the whole estate and she still looks absolutely ravishing. I shall stay on myself, till I die. It's wicked that everyone shouldn't feel like that.'

Barbara Cartland, best-selling author, and still going strong in her eighties

'You have one body, and it's up to you to take care of it. It makes even greater sense to take greater care, the older you get, of your bones and your muscles. You can exercise the way I do, with music, if that's what you enjoy; you can go to a local sports centre, you can swim, check your posture, be aware of breathing – deep breathing, not short, shallow breaths – low-fat and high-fibre diet, chuck out the frying pan, grill and trim meat so that there's no fat on it, plenty of fruit and vegetables, lots of yoghurt, lots of low-fat cheese and skimmed milk.

I'm forty now, and as I approach the menopause I'm looking at the various symptoms I might come across. And as a patron of the National Osteoporosis Society, I see many of the sufferers from this particularly unpleasant old-age disease in women. HRT helps with so many symptoms of the menopause that when the time comes I'll be the first to take it.

Lizzie Webb, exercise star of TV AM

'A crippling disease in early childhood left me with complex lower-limb joint problems, which were exacerbated by the onset of osteo-arthritis in my mid-forties. Through my work as a journalist, I was lucky enough to meet and be taken on as a patient by a research rheumatologist with a major interest in HRT. I was put on that treatment, both to manage my menopause and to protect against osteoporosis which, in my condition, would have been even more disastrous than it usually is.

I have been on HRT now for fifteen years and its effectiveness against normal menopause problems was always quite obvious. I also felt it gave me the energy and drive needed to cope with a demanding job, with some inevitable pain from my arthritis, and from the hip-replacement operations that became necessary as I grew older.

Recently, at the age of sixty-five, I had to have a hip replacement *re-done*, an operation where good results are by no means guaranteed because the state of the bone can be suspect. In my own case, not only was the operation successful, with a better and quicker recovery than I have ever made before, but the surgeon remarked to me afterwards on the strength of the bones and the marked absence of any sign of osteoporosis. This literally "inside" information confirmed for me that HRT had been doing the job of protecting my bones extremely well. I do wish more women would realize how important it is to get on to HRT early, particularly if, for some reason, like me, they can only take very limited exercise.'

Ms Bobby Freeman, journalist and food writer,
Newport

Other well-known women publicized as using HRT include: Margaret Thatcher, Cleo Laine, Diana Rigg, Valerie Singleton, Sue Lawley, Dora Bryan and Gloria Hunniford. Also, at a time when it was far more difficult for women in the public eye to discuss such matters, Jean Kent, Barbara Cartland and Barbara Kelly bravely described how HRT had helped them, in the first edition of *No Change*, published in 1975. They helped to lead the way.

Appendix 2

Statements and quotes from doctors

'The menopause and the years that follow can be regarded as biological sabotage on hitherto healthy women. The three most important long-term problems that result from this are those relating to depression, heart attacks and osteoporosis, and oestrogen has markedly beneficial effects on them all.

All women experience progressive loss of body collagen after the menopause, which produces thin, dry skin, brittle nails, aching of muscles and bones and loss of the collagen connective tissue matrix of bone. It is this change which is the fundamental cause of osteoporosis, because the collagen 'scaffolding' is lost and the bone mineral disappears, leaving bone strength greatly diminished.

Even by the age of sixty, one woman in four suffers an osteoporotic fracture and the cost in human and financial terms of the broken hips, collapsed spines and fractured wrists is quite simply appalling.

There is no doubt that these changes are preventable by oestrogen replacement therapy and there is also evidence emerging that bone tissue can be replaced even in the severely osteoporotic skeleton by routes of therapy such as implants, which produce a higher oestradiol level.

Costs for hospital charges alone to deal with osteoporosis are now estimated at £800 million a year. That fact that it is so expensive is the only good thing about osteoporosis, because it means that the logic for availability of HRT for *prevention* of bone disease and other menopause problems is becoming overwhelming even to the most ungenerous of paymasters.

We have to decide whether to offer oestrogen therapy to all women of the appropriate age or just to target high-risk groups. As the long-term *Leisure World* study from California has clearly shown that oestrogen therapy produces an *extra four years of life*, probably good years, it does not make much sense to ration oestrogen therapy in this way. It is rather like insisting that special people can have clean water but the rest of us have to use the village pond.

Withholding HRT doesn't make economic sense, either. A woman could be kept well and her bones protected for one or two years for what it would cost to carry out a single proper screening test.'

John Studd, Consultant Gynaecologist, King's College Hospital

'Prevention of osteoporosis is certainly high among the many known benefits of Hormone Replacement Therapy. Nothing in life is completely risk-free, but the risks of HRT (both known and hypothetical) are livable with and more than outweighed by the benefits for most women.

As a result, it is my opinion that HRT should not be restricted to those women who happen to get hot flushes or similar symptoms just around the time of the menopause. There should be serious consideration of this treatment for *all* women and one really needs a reason for *not* giving it. The reason could be that she is unlikely to develop osteoporosis by virtue of her body mass or racial characteristics, or that she simply chooses to let nature take its course. But for many other women the *option* of obtaining the known long-

term benefits of this treatment should not be withheld from them, as it sometimes is at present.'
John Guillebaud, Medical Director, Margaret Pyke Centre

'In 1972, when I was first involved in a menopause clinic, the major emphasis of treatment was to relieve acute symptoms such as flushes, sweats, insomnia and vaginal dryness. Treatment was aimed at giving the lowest therapeutic doses for a short period of time, varying between six and twenty-four months.

Since then, there has been a marked shift in our attitude toward what we are treating and for how long. The long-term effects of oestrogen depletion are osteoporosis and cardio-vascular disease. Both can be significantly helped by administration of oesotrogens, particularly osteoporosis, and my advice to patients is that they should continue therapy from the start of menopausal symptoms until they are at least sixty. In practice, many patients will continue for longer.

Those that we are particularly keen to treat are women with an early menopause, who are thin, fair and who smoke. Our own research project into vertebral bone loss strongly supports the contention that long-term oestrogen therapy is beneficial in the prevention of bone loss.'
Peter Bowen-Simpkins, Consultant Gynaecologist, Singleton Hospital, Swansea

'Osteoporosis poses an under-recognized threat to all women. Most do not consider the problems of old age to be a matter of concern until they are approaching the age of retirement, but the prevention of osteoporosis begins much earlier. It begins in childhood with a good diet and plenty of exercise during the growth of the skeleton. At midlife, when bone loss begins, we need to recognize those women most at risk of future osteoporosis and counsel them about prevention with Hormone Replacement Therapy or, if this is contra-indicated, other alternatives.

At present, measuring bone mass is the best way of finding out who is at greatest risk and this gives them a more definite reason to take HRT for five or more years.

Hopefully, bone-mass measurement will become available in all parts of the United Kingdom, but, for this approach to be effective, the public and doctors must be made aware of osteoporosis, its consequences and ways of preventing it. Books like this are an important way of increasing the awareness of this enormous problem.'

Anthony D. Woolf, Consultant Rheumatologist, Royal Cornwall Hospital, Truro, Cornwall

'A strong plea can be made for HRT as preventive therapy for women over forty-five, not only with a view to the prevention of climacteric complaints, but also to facilitating her adaptation to her new social roles by bringing – or keeping – the woman in the optimum condition, thus enabling her to cope adequately with social adjustments.

The treatable and preventable complaints are the following: (1) the majority of manifestations of the climacteric; (2) atrophy of the vaginal wall and related complaints; (3) skin atrophy; (4) incontinence of the ageing woman; and, (5) osteoporosis.'

Dr P. A. Van Keep, International Health Foundation, Geneva, Switzerland

'It is important to decide whether one should aim at prophylaxis or treatment. By the time one treats osteoporosis, for example, a considerable amount of bone has already been lost. It is a case of shutting the stable door after the horse has gone. It is not quite the same as treating the atrophic vagina. Even after this has developed, one can get a good and quick reversal with oestrogens. The practice of medicine, as a whole, tends nowadays to be more and more a prophylactic type of medicine. I do not think we should treat a condition when it arises, we should think more about *prevention*. That is why I would argue strongly in favour of replacement therapy in connection with bone disease.'

J. C. Gallagher, MRC Mineral Metabolism Unit,
General Infirmary, Leeds

'Nature condemns women to a biological castration in middle life. With the loss of the female hormones come many threats to their wellbeing and health. Dominant among the long-term effects of the menopause is weakness of the skeleton, osteoporosis. One in four women in this country will eventually suffer an osteoporosis-related fracture. But post-menopausal osteoporosis is a *preventable* condition not yet being prevented. One doctor has said that if men suffered a similar fate, something would have been done about it long ago.

For women, that something is available *now* – Hormone Replacement Therapy (HRT). It may not be the answer for every woman. Health-screening techniques are still not sharp enough to predict with certainty which one in every four women will, and which three out of four will not, get osteoporosis if nothing is done. But this is not the only consideration. The benefits of HRT are now seen to include not only the prevention of osteoporosis but a reduction in the risk of heart attacks and strokes, with studies concluding that it leads to an increased expectation of life.

Of course, controversies go on about whether or not the risks of certain cancers will be raised (most of the evidence is that they are not), but while doctors argue about these, the frequency of osteoporotic hip fractures is increasing faster than the number of elderly in the population would predict, and HRT remains so far the only practical method of preventing them.'

> *Allan Dixon, Consultant Physician, Royal National Hospital, Bath, and Chairman of the National Osteoporosis Society*

'Some of the women who come to our menopause clinics are very unhappy – some of them think they're going mad, and after a few months on HRT you see that this same person regains confidence and is much happier and coping with life much better.

It worries me that there are many thousands of women in similar circumstances, who are just having to carry on suffering because they have not had HRT. I would never try to force it on anybody, but I do genuinely think that all women should be given the opportunity of having hormone replacement, the same way as all diabetics should be able to get insulin.

As regards risks, they are very small – someone who smokes is doing something far more dangerous than taking hormone replacement. If you think of people who die as a result of alcohol in road traffic accidents, or from cirrhosis of the liver – then alcohol too is more dangerous than HRT.

I genuinely believe the risks are far less than the benefits, such as the protection HRT gives against osteoporosis and against heart disease and strokes. If all ladies who wanted Hormone Replacement Therapy were given it, then the total saving in lives would be greater than any extra loss.'

> *Dr David McKay, Consultant Gynaecologist, Bone Metabolism Research Unit, Western Infirmary and Stobhill Hospital, Glasgow*

'All women who suffer from menopausal symptoms should be treated and not just reassured or tranquillized. I would like to see long-term replacement therapy, using natural oestrogen, available for all who want it and I feel women should be rising up in a body and asking for this treatment.'

Audrey Midwinter, Consultant Gynaecologist, Bristol

'I still feel very saddened at the number of women with miserable menopausal problems who are being denied HRT at a time in their lives when they need all the help they can get. Both women and some doctors have been unnecessarily alarmed by reported complications in HRT which have now been resolved by modern prescribing techniques.

There is no doubt in selected patients oestrogen can transform the life of the woman and her family, and offer her protection against osteoporosis, strokes and heart disease in future years. It is the right of every woman who feels she will benefit from this treatment to have an *informed and unbiased* opinion from a member of the medical profession.'

J. A. Jordan, Consultant Gynaecologist, Birmingham and Midland Hospital for Women

'We know of one way, and only one, of preventing post-menopausal bone loss, and that is Hormone Replacement Therapy. To identify women at highest risk and most in need of this treatment, we have developed a simple biochemical test. In a recent study we showed that this test, involving only one blood sample and one urine sample, plus measurement of height and weight, could correctly identify seventy-nine per cent of fast bone losers, and seventy-eight per cent of slow bone losers.

Used for preliminary screening this would allow the majority of post-menopausal women at risk of osteoporosis to be identified at reasonable cost and early in the post-menopausal period, *before* bone mineral content has fallen substantially.'

Claus Christiansen, Department of Clinical Chemistry, University of Copenhagen and Department of Clinical Physiology, Aalborg Hospital, Denmark

'If replacement therapy is commenced at the time of the menopause and continued for five years, it's been estimated that a patient's risk of femoral neck fracture will be halved, and even greater protection may be afforded by longer-term therapy. Weight-bearing exercise may help prevent post-menopausal bone loss in the femoral neck, but should be advised in addition, rather than as an alternative, to oestrogen therapy.

Calcium supplements do not appear to prevent bone loss in post-menopausal women and need not be prescribed as an adjunct to HRT. Other drugs such as calcitonin, or disphosonates show promise as alternatives to oestrogen, but further work is necessary before their use can be recommended for prevention of osteoporosis.'

Michael Cust, Research Fellow in Gynaecology, Cavendish Clinic, London

'Osteoporosis is a major threat to women's health and, despite all the publicity, hip fractures seem to be increasing. Women of all ages should be aware of the problem and use every opportunity to question health professionals. Altering people's lifestyles is a daunting task, and GPs can at times be overwhelmed by demands on their time, but a few words of advice can always be fitted into even the busiest surgery.

Preventing osteoporosis in the long term requires lifelong surveillance and expertise to give proper continuity of care. This is best achieved in general practice, but midwives, health visitors, district and practice nurses can also be approached at different stages of life. Health education in schools is very important. From nursery school onwards, the principles involved in maintaining good strong bones need to be taught, in particular the value of exercise.

Adult women need also to recognize that exercise is for life, that the Pill *probably* protects their bones, and that for the older woman HRT *definitely* does and is available on the NHS. Perhaps the most important fact to realize is that prevention of osteoporosis rests almost entirely in a woman's own hands.'

Dr Christina Kennaway, GP, Bath

'Osteoporotic fracture represents a major challenge to public health. At least one in three women will sustain an osteoporotic fracture within her lifetime. The most serious of these is fracture of the hip, which induces a great deal of permanent disability and, particularly in the elderly, is a significant contributory cause of death. The occurrence of hip fracture and indeed all other osteoporotic fractures is increasing. This is in part due to the increased life-expectancy and longevity of the population, but over and above this there is an increase in age- and sex-specific rates, perhaps related to our more sedentary lifestyle. If the current rate of increase continues unabated, then predictions suggest that the occurrence of hip fractures in this country will double by the year 2016.

The treatment of reduced bone density poses many problems. The rebuilding of the skeleton is a much more difficult task than the prevention of bone loss. There have been considerable advances in our understanding of the way in which loss can be prevented. Hormone Replacement Therapy certainly prevents bone loss, but there are a number of other treatments which are available or being tested which are capable of preventing or delaying the rate of bone loss. The availability of these treatments means that strategies

need to be developed to identify women, particularly at the time of the menopause, who are at greatest risk from future osteoporotic fracture. Accurate and precise methods have been developed for measuring bone density, but are not widely available. One of the priorities of the immediate future is to develop facilities for screening so that women concerned about their skeletal status can have an accurate estimate of their future risk, and on the basis of this decide whether or not to accept preventative measures.'
John A. Kanis, Consultant Physician, Medical School,
University of Sheffield

'Accurate prediction of the likelihood that an individual will develop osteoporosis is a desired goal for two reasons. First, there are no safe, highly effective methods to treat *existing* osteoporosis; to restore bone tissue to an already osteoporotic skeleton. Second, by contrast, preventative strategies to reduce post-menopausal and ageing-associated bone loss in some subjects *are* available through oestrogen therapy and calcitonin.

Oestrogen therapy has been demonstrated in both prospective as well as case-control studies to be the most effective way to reduce the rate of post-menopausal bone loss and to prevent fractures.

Calcitonin too reduces bone loss and is an alternative in high-risk subjects who are not candidates for oestrogen replacement. It also has an analgesic effect in patients with the crush-fracture syndrome. For the moment its high cost, parenteral route of administration (injection) and uncertain long-term effectiveness limit its applicability.

Increasing calcium intake to acceptable bone protection levels is also recommended; current evidence points to a requirement of 1000 milligrams a day for adults and 1500 milligrams a day for post-menopausal women and others at high risk of osteoporosis.

In addition, physical exercise of an anti-gravity nature (weight-bearing) may well promote skeletal density during the maturing years and reduce aging-associated losses.'

Dr William A. Peck, Professor of Medicine,
Washington University, USA

'Osteoporosis is an extremely difficult disease to treat and the only future lies in the *prevention* of bone loss. At the present time the only safe, established method for achieving this is Hormone Replacement Therapy, but I do share some concern about possible breast cancer risk with long-term use. I do not, therefore, favour a blanket policy of long-term HRT for *all* women. I believe that those at greatest risk of developing osteoporosis require to take oestrogen, and the arguments centre around how best to identify these women.

It is now well established that the single best predictor of subsequent osteoporosis is bone-mineral measurement and with the new generation machines, i.e. dual energy X-ray absorptiometry, it is now a simple matter to measure bone density in the clinically relevant sites of spine and femur.

Ideally, women should have bone-mass measurements carried out at the time of the menopause and those with good normal results can be reassured. Those with low values require HRT. There will inevitably be a 'grey area' and perhaps those women need to have bone-mass measurements repeated in several years' time to assess the amount of loss that has occurred over that period.

I am an advocate of screening for osteoporosis, as the only alternative is long-term HRT for all. Unfortunately, routine screening is not feasible with the facilities presently available, and I would suggest that several centres are funded to investigate further ways and means.'

Ignac Fogelman, Consultant Physician, Guy's Hospital, London

'Post-menopausal osteoporosis is the most common metabolic bone disease in the Western world. Only recently, however, has the extent of the problem come to be recognized. Two factors have contributed to this. First, our understanding of the disease has now expanded as a result of new and sophisticated techniques for measuring bone mass and the hormones that regulate it. Second, the expansion of the post-menopausal population, which comprises around sixteen per cent of our total population, has led to ever-increasing numbers of cases. The average woman today can expect to spend almost a third of her life in the post-menopausal state.

HRT is the only way to stop post-menopausal bone loss and, if it's introduced soon after the onset of the menopause, the bones will not get thin enough to fracture. This prevention of osteoporosis is all-important, as once bone is lost it's difficult, if not impossible, to restore. The best one can hope is to prevent further loss.

But, however desirable it may be, it's still not possible to impose preventive treatment on all post-menopausal women. Some women and even some doctors may subscribe to the view that the menopause is 'natural', but certainly the development of osteoporosis is not. Women should thus be made aware of the risks of the menopause and all should have access to HRT.

The earlier the menopause and the longer a woman spends in the post-menopausal state, the greater are her chances of developing brittle bones and fractures. For example, I have seen osteoporosis in a girl of twenty-nine years because she underwent her natural menopause prematurely at age seventeen. Thus, women who experience their menopause before forty, or perhaps even forty-five years of age should be regarded as at particularly high risk. Because the post-menopausal ovary still makes a small contribution to the overall oestrogen status, where a woman has to have them removed and there is no contribution at all, preventive treatment in the form of HRT is mandatory. It should also be remembered that hysterectomy alone may sometimes compromise ovarian function.

Women who have had periods of amenorrhoea, for whatever reason, are also likely to have thinner bones by the time they reach the menopause and they too should be considered at special risk.

Conversely, pregnancy and oral contraceptive use should be regarded as beneficial factors. Both help to maintain whatever peak adult bone mass has been genetically determined. Because genetic factors are so important in relation to potential bone mass, a family history of osteoporosis can also indicate increased risk and should provide motivation for acceptance of preventive therapy.

In my view, despite the still widespread use of calcium and Vitamin D preparations, there is no convincing evidence of them being an effective alternative to HRT. Calcitonin may be if problems over route of administration and expense can be resolved. Bisphosphonates are also a potential alternative and further research is awaited.

Where anabolic steroids and fluoride are concerned, although both have potent effects on the skeleton, side-effects preclude their general usage. HRT currently remains the most effective method of preventing osteoporosis and fractures.'

John C. Stevenson, Consultant Endocrinologist, Wynn Institute for Metabolic Research, London

'Something like one post-menopausal women in four suffers to a greater or less extent from osteoporosis, for which properly prescribed HRT is a reliably effective prophylaxis. Although etidronate is now being claimed to have preventative as well as curative value for this condition, it cannot, of course, relieve the other symptoms directly due to oestrogen deficiency, and nor is there reason to believe it can reduce the incidence of cardio- or cerebro-vascular disease as oestrogens are known to do.'

Gerald Swyer, Chairman, Women's Health Concern;
Formerly Consultant Endocrinologist, University
College Hospital, London

'In the whole of nature only the human female experiences a menopause. While other animals remain potentially fertile until death, the woman of today, with a life expectancy of about seventy-eight years, will spend an average of one-third of her life after the cessation of reproductive potential, in a state of ovarian failure and oestrogen deficiency.

Fortunately, the effects of hormone deficiency are easily corrected by Hormone Replacement Therapy (HRT), and the eradication of the acute symptoms of hot flushes, night sweats, lethargy, dry vagina, etc., can be very dramatic and a rewarding experience for the woman, her family and the prescribing doctor.

However, although these symptoms can significantly lower the quality of life, they are not life-threatening and no one has ever died from a hot flush. But the long-term effects of oestrogen deficiency such as osteoporosis may result in fractures which are definitely life-threatening. Fracture of the hip is associated with fifteen to twenty per cent mortality and half of those who survive do not return to an independent existence.

For the long-term health of women, it is imperative that the value of HRT in preventing osteoporosis is more widely appreciated. Unfortunately, all too often the communication of medical matters to the lay public is either ill-informed, sensationalized or misleading. Hopefully, this book by a journalist, so well respected by the medical profession that she is frequently invited to talk at medical meetings, will stimulate much wider usage of HRT to help preserve the long-term quality of life for women.'

David Sturdee, Consultant Gynaecologist and Director of the Menopause Clinic, Solihull Hospital

'GPs are very aware of the suffering caused by osteoporosis in older women. Prevention at last appears to be possible and the experience we have gained over the years in prescribing HRT to relieve the more obvious menopause symptoms means we are now ideally placed to implement its prophylactic use to help protect against osteoporosis.

Well-Woman Clinics in the practice setting are rapidly becoming universal, combining routine breast and cervical smear screening with measurements and recording of other parameters of health. This, together with increasing use of computers, means that all women can be offered regular screening. These clinics provide an excellent opportunity for HRT counselling as the menopause approaches, for identifying risk factors for osteoporosis and discussing treatment, as well as for regular monitoring of patients once HRT has been started.

Our patients' greatest reservations concern the long-term safety of HRT, particularly with regard to breast cancer. GPs look forward to the reassurance of large long-term studies to discount these fears and to combat the often ill-informed interpretations of medical reports in the lay Press.'

Mark Vernon-Roberts, General Practitioner, Swansea

'On the whole, general practitioners are the best people to manage the menopause. They know the patient's previous history and her social and psychological problems. This helps in the diagnosis of her presenting symptoms and makes preliminary screening much easier. General practitioners need to agree with the local gynaecologist on which patients to investigate and when. However, they need training in the diagnosis, screening and supervision of patients. This is now available in a new folder on Hormone Replacement Therapy from the Royal College of General Practitioners.

Many women are reluctant to take hormones because of embarking on 'periods' again. The doctor needs to be aware of their feelings and to be able to discuss the pros and cons of treatments so that the patient is involved in the decision-making process. Many are anxious about a possible increase in the risk of breast cancer and mammography screening is advisable before and at intervals during treatment.

HRT is now reasonably safe as long as patients are properly supervised and long-term treatment offers protection to the bones and the heart. Many more women would benefit from it if their doctors had the confidence to offer such screening and supervision.

My personal view of HRT has swung over the years from cautious scepticism to acceptance and now to enthusiasm. Unlike the event on the road to Damascus my personal conversion has taken place over a period and is based on the scientific evidence which has emerged in that time.

In our practice clinic, we now actively contact women and encourage them to embark on HRT and a range of preventive measures which have been shown experimentally to reduce the incidence of osteoporosis. An account of this clinic has been accepted for publication in the *British Journal of General Practitioners*.'

Jean Coope, General Practitioner, Macclesfield

'Until recently we have had no real answer to osteo-porosis except to encourage women in their middle years to be as physically active as possible. Only by using the skeleton vigorously during the reproductive years will many women be able to build up a "calcium bank" in their long bones that will see them through the calcium-losing years ahead.

Two great steps forward have been HRT and, more recently, calcitonin. HRT dramatically stops the calcium loss, makes most women feel much better, and is largely without risk if care is taken to exclude women with a high risk of breast cancer. This is not because it will induce breast cancer in such women, but because if one should arise, it would be difficult not to blame HRT for the condition. If anything, evidence strongly suggests that far from inducing cancers, HRT may well prevent them – especially of the ovary and uterus.

However, HRT is not normally available to women with known breast disease and until now they have had to make do with calcium supplements and extra Vitamin D. Neither has been proved to be of benefit. The news that calcitonin may soon be available should encourage them. It stops the breakdown of bone calcium and turns the balance towards restoring bone strength to the levels of a younger age. I look forward to many of my patients carrying with them a convenient calcitonin spray – along with their lipsticks and perfume in their handbags.

Meanwhile, exercise for all is the thing – everyone should be physically active, before and after the meno-pause.'

Dr Tom Smith, Specialist in Pharmaceutical Medicine

'Over the last ten to fifteen years, major advances have been made in our understanding of both the short- and long-term sequelae of oestrogen deprivation at the menopause. There is overwhelming evidence that HRT is not only the best treatment for distressing meno-pausal symptoms, but also our only means of preventing osteoporosis and its tragic consequences. Perhaps even more important than this, however, we know that oestrogen replacement has a significant role to play in the prevention of arterial disease in women, reducing substantially the number of deaths from heart attacks and strokes. Arterial disease is the major cause of death amongst women in this country, outnumbering deaths from cancer of the breast, uterus and ovary combined. Thus HRT has the potential to make an enormous positive impact on women's health, both for individuals and for society as a whole.

There is a growing awareness amongst the general public that the problems of the menopause are considerable, but can be overcome by the provision of HRT under medical supervision. Specialists agree that the benefits of such therapy far outweigh the risks, but many members of the medical profession are yet to be convinced. As we move into the 1990s, it is important that research into new forms of treatment continues but, at the same time, up-to-date information must be disseminated to all health care professionals, if we are to take advantage of the golden opportunity that HRT can bring.'

Malcolm Whitehead, Lecturer in Obstetrics and Gynaecology, King's College Hospital Medical School

Appendix 3

National osteoporosis survey, 1990

Method

A questionnaire was sent to all 10,000 members of the NOS and elicited a seventy-five per cent response. All replies are being computerized and the following extracts are from the first 1000 run through for surnames A to E. The NOS recognize that results from this self-selected sample cannot be extrapolated to the general population. Nevertheless some of the information is interesting, even startling.

Extracts from preliminary findings

1. Replies revealed sixty-one per cent of members had already been diagnosed as suffering from osteoporosis.
2. Average age of sufferers was only sixty.
3. Thirty-three per cent of sufferers had a family history of osteoporosis.
4. Twenty-three per cent had had either hysterectomy or oophorectomy – over half of them before age forty-seven.
5. Ninety-eight per cent of these had never received HRT.
6. Of oophorectomized sufferers only 0.6 per cent had had HRT.
7. Of *all* sufferers only 3.6 per cent had received HRT.

8. Two per cent had been on high doses of cortico-steroid for over six months.
9. 4.5 per cent had suffered from thyroid disease.
10. Ten per cent of sufferers had had dentures fitted under the age of thirty and this offers an interesting area for further research to see if early dental decay is an indicator of bone problems.
11. The preliminary findings also showed that where women are given HRT, they are not remaining on treatment long enough for it to have any significant effect on bone mass.
12. The reason for coming off HRT is usually 'on doctor's advice'!

NOS suggestions for urgent action

• Every woman who now has an oophorectomy should be offered HRT and this should be monitored to ensure she does not discontinue treatment for some minor reason. It is important that the right product be found to suit the patient. The NOS is currently preparing a second booklet for doctors, giving more details on the side-effects of HRT and how varying doses and types of HRT can be used to find the right individual prescription.

• Every woman who has a hysterectomy should be considered for HRT. If she does not have it, she should be closely monitored.

• All women who have had an oophorectomy in the past should be recalled to consider HRT before it is too late. The same applies to women who have had an early natural menopause. It should be automatic to consider these women for Hormone Replacement Therapy.

It is estimated that two million women in this country suffer from osteoporosis. If, as in the sample, fourteen per cent of them developed the condition following hysterectomy or oophorectomy, then gynaecologists have it in their power to save over a quarter of a million women from osteoporosis by following through their work on the operating table. By taking responsibility for compensating a woman for her loss of oestrogen after surgery, enormous savings could be made in human suffering and NHS costs.

In human terms it would mean extending the normal life and saving from terrible pain, deformity and loss of independence, hundreds of thousands of women like the NOS members listed here as typical examples from the first 1000 replies analysed:

Mrs D of Wales with five fractures at fifty-five after an oophorectomy and no HRT;

Mrs E of Surrey with five fractures at sixty-four after hysterectomy at forty-three;

Mrs E of Merseyside with three fractures and severe height loss at seventy after hysterectomy at forty-eight;

Mrs E of Leicester with a curved spine and height loss at only fifty-five, after oophorectomy at forty;

Mrs R of Hertfordshire with two fractures at sixty-five after hysterectomy at forty-one;

Mrs E of Yorkshire with five fractures at fifty-six after an oophorectomy at thirty-seven.

All of this small random group, extracted from the 1000 sample analysed, replied on their questionnaire that they wished they had had the option of Hormone Replacement Therapy when their surgery was carried out. The NOS strongly suggests that while debate may continue about other risk factors for osteoporosis and about how many of the general population should be considered for HRT, *all* women who have ever had an early oophorectomy, hysterectomy or early natural menopause should be urgently identified and considered for HRT *now*, before the end of 1990, and before they too succumb to osteoporosis.

Linda Edwards, The Director, National Osteoporosis Society

General references

Coope, J., Roberts, D., 'A Clinic for the prevention of osteoporosis in general practice' (*British Journal of General Practice*. (1990), 4C, 336)

Coope, J., *Hormone Replacement Therapy* (Royal College General Practitioners, 1990)

Gambrel, R. D., 'Hormone Replacement Therapy and breast cancer' (Maturitas 9, (1987), 123–133)

Henderson, B. E., et al., 'Oestrogen use and cardiovascular disease', (*American Journal of Obstetrics and Gynaecology* 154 (1986), 1181–1186)

Lindsay, R., 'Managing Osteoporosis: current trends, future possibilities' (*Geriatrics* (1987), 42, 35–41)

Lindsay, R., and Saitken, J. M. et al., 'Long-term prevention of post-menopausal osteoporosis by oestrogen' (*Lancet* 1, 1038–40)

Padwick, M., and Whitehead M., 'Oestrogen Deficiency: Causes, consequences and management' (August 1985, 275–284)

Rauramo, L., 'A review of study findings of the risks and benefits of oestrogen therapy' (Maturitas 8, (1986), 177–187)

Riis, B. J., and Christiansen, C., 'Prevention of post-menopausal bone loss: effects of alternative forms of oestrogens, alternative oestrogens and calcium addition' (NucCompact 18, (1987), 24–28)

Stevenson J.C. (Ed), New Techniques in Metabolic Bone Disease (Wright, 1990)

Whitehead, Sichella, and Van Keep, *The Climacteric and Beyond* (Pantheon Publishing, 1987)

Woolfe, A. D., and A. Dixon, *Osteoporosis: A Clinical Guide* (Dunitz, 1988)

'NIH Osteoporosis Consensus Conference', *British Medical Journal*, 1987 (914–916)

'The Framingham Study', *New England Journal of Medicine*, 1985 (313, 1044–9)

Medical references

Chapter 1

1. Beringer, R. T. O., McSherry, D. M. G. G., and Taggart, H. McA. (Christiansen Ed., 1985). Osteoporosis Proceedings of the Copenhagen International Symposium.
2. Padwick, M., and Whitehead, M. (Update, August 1985: 275–284). Raurama, I. (Maturitas 8 (1986), 177–187).

Chapter 2

1. Rigitti, B. A., Nussbaum, S. R., et al (*New England Journal of Medicine* 311 (1984), 1401–6). Trave, J. Fogelman, I., et al (*British Medical Journal* 295 (1987), 474–5).
2. See reference 1, Chapter One, above.
3. Knowelden, J., et al (*Preventative and Social Medicine* 18 (1974), 130).
   Owen, R. A., et al (*Clinical Orthopaedics and Related Research* 150 (1980), 172).
   Newton-John, F. H. and Morgan, D. B. (*Clinical Orthopaedics and Related Research* 71 (1970), 229–252).

Chapter 3

1. Smith, D.M. et al, (*Journal of Clinical Investigation* (1973)).
2. Daniell, H. W. (*Journal of the American Medical Association* 221 (1972), 509). Baron, J. A.,

'Smoking and Reproductive Health' (PSGG Publishing (1987), Massachusetts). Lindquist, O., and Bengtesson, C., (Maturitas 1 (1979), 171).

3. Aitken, J. M., Hart D. M., and Lindsay, R. (*British Medical Journal* 3 (1973), 515–8). Baber, R., Abdalla, H., and Studd, J., *Progress in Obstetrics and Gynaecology* (Churchill, 1988).

4. Spector, T. D. (*British Medical Journal* 200 (1989), 1434–5).

Chapter 4

1. Nordin, B. E. C., and Gallagher, J. C. (*The Lancet* 1 (1972), 503). Nordin, B. E. C., and Gallagher, J. C. (*Clinical Endocrinology* 1 (1972), 57). Nordin, B. E. C. (*British Medical Journal* 1 (1971), 571).

2. Aitken, J. M., Hart, D. M., Lindsay, R. (*British Medical Journal* 3 (1977), 571).

3. Gordan, C. S. (*American Family Physician* 8 (1973), 6, 74).

Chapter 5

1. Lindsay, R., Hart D. M., et al (*Clinical Science and Molecular Medicine* 54 (1977), 193–5).

2. Smith D. C., (*New England Journal of Medicine* 293 (1975) 1164).

3. Sturdee, D. W., Wade-Evans, and Studd, J. W. W. (*British Journal of Obstetrics and Gynaecology* 84 (1977), 193–5). Campbell, S., et al (*Post-graduate Medical Journal* 54, supplement 2 (1978), 59–64). Sturdee D. W., Paterson, M. E. L., et al (*British Medical Journal* (1978), 1575–7).

4. Whitehead M. I. (*Acta Obstetrics and Gynaecology* 134, (1986), 81–91).

5. Paterson, M. E. L., Sturdee, D., Thom, M., and Studd, J. W. W. (*British Medical Journal 1* (1980), 822–4).

6. Rauramo, L., (Maturitas 9 (1986), 77–187).
7. European Organization for Cancer Prevention & Studies, in *European Journal of Obstetrics and Gynaecology and Reproductive Biology* 26 (1987), 6).
8. Brinton, L. A., Hoover, R. N., Szklo M., et al (*Cancer* 47 (1981), 2523). Brinton, L. A., Hoover, R. N., and Fraumeni J. F. (*Journal of the American Medical Association* 252 (1986) 63–69). Bergkrst, L., et al (*New England Journal of Medicine* 321 (1986) 293–297).
9. Gambrell, R. D. (*Obstetrics and Gynaecology* 62 (1983), 438–443). Gambrell, R. D., (*International Journal of Fertility* 31 (1986), 112–122). Wingo, P. A., et al. (*Journal of the American Medical Association* 257 (1987), 209–215).
10. Hunt, K., Vessey, M., McPherson, K., and Coleman, M. (*British Journal of Obstetrics and Gynaecology* 94 (1987), 620–635).
11. Montgomery, J. C., Studd, J. W. W., et al (*The Lancet* 1 (1988), 297).
12. Studd, J. W. W., Savvas, M., and Johnson, M. (*The Lancet* 1 (1989), 339).
13. Burk, T. L., and Barrett-Connor, E. (*Epidemiological Reviews* 7 (1985), 80–104). Kaplan, M. M., (*Journal of Reproductive Medicine* 30 (1985), 802–804).
   Henderson, B. C., et al (*American Journal of Obstetrics and Gynaecology* 154 (1986), 1181–1186).
   Colditzs, G. A., et al (*New England Journal of Medicine* 316 (1987), 1103–1110).
14. Oliver, M. F., and Boyd, G. S. (*The Lancet* 1 (1959) 690).
15. Brincat, M., Moniz, C. F., Studd, J. W. W., et al (*British Medical Journal* 287 (1983), 1337–1338). Punnonen, R., et al (Maturitas 5 (1984), 259).

16.   Report, Aalberg Conference (*British Medical Journal* 295 (1987), 914–915).

Chapter 6

1.   Shapira D. (*Journal of the Royal Society of Medicine* 81 (1988), 461–3).
2.   Chaw, R., Harrison, J. E., and Notarius, C., (*British Medical Journal* 295 (1987), 1441–1444).
3.   Ettinger, B., Genant, H. K., and Cann, C. E. (*Annual of International Medicine* 106 (1987), 40–453).
4.   Editorial, (*The Lancet* 1 (1987), 306–307). Chalmers, J. and Ho, K. C. (*Journal of Bone and Joint Surgery* 52B (1970), 667–675).

Chapter 7

1.   Selby, P. L., et al (*Clinical Science* 69 (1985), 265–271).
2.   Woolfe, A. D., and Dixon, A. St. J. (*Osteoporosis: A Clinical Guide*, Dunitz, 1988).

Chapter 8

1.   Sturdee, D. W., Wade-Evans, Studd, J. (*British Journal of Obstetrics and Gynaecology* 84 (1977), 193–5). Sturdee, D. W., Paterson, M. E. L., et al (*British Medical Journal* 1 (1979) 11575–7).
2.   Lane, G., Siddle, N. C., Whitehead, M. I., et al (*British Journal of Obstetrics and Gynaecology* 93 (1986), 55–62).
3.   Fletcher, C. A., et al (*Acta Endocrinological* 117 (Copenhagen, 1988) 339–342).
4.   Storm, J., Thorsburg G, et al (*New England Journal of Medicine* 322 (1990), 1265–71).
5.   Christiansen, C., Christiansen M. S., et al (*The Lancet* 1 (1981), 459–461.
     Lindsay, R., Hart, D. M., and Aitken, J. M. (*The Lancet* 1 (1976), 1038–1040).

Munk-Jenson, et al (*British Medical Journal* 296 (1988), 1150–1152).
Studd, J. W. W., and Fogelman, I. (1990).
6. Christiansen, C., et al (*The Lancet* 1 (16 May 1987), 1105–1108).

Helpful agencies

Women's Health Concern
83 Earl's Court Road, London W8 6EP (071 938 3932)

As Women's Health Care, this was the first organization dedicated to educating and advising women on the menopause and to steering them toward appropriate help and treatment.

It was set up in 1972 as a non-profitmaking charitable trust. In recent years, under the name of Women's Health Concern, Founder Coordinator, Joan Jenkins, and Dr Gerald Swyer, the eminent consultant endocrinologist who chairs the Medical Advisory Board, have together extended the scope of WHC work to cover a wide range of gynaecological conditions.

During the two years from 1987 to 1989, WHC doctors and counsellors dealt voluntarily with more than 130,000 inquiries from women who had failed to get satisfactory answers elsewhere. Of these, sixty-seven per cent were concerned with the menopause and HRT.

Special WHC leaflets are free to anyone who writes in with an SAE. The original objective of advancing health education among women has been extended recently into professional areas, with the organization of Medical Symposia, special nurses' study days and one-week courses for nurse counsellors.

The workload carried by WHC is recognized in grants from the Department of Health towards administrative expenses, now increased from £21,000 a year to £45,000 for a special three-year project involving new pilot counselling schemes. The Department of Social Security has also donated £10,000 toward WHC counselling services in England and an appeal has been launched for the further £500,000 needed to cover the costs of expanding these services throughout England and Wales, and enabling Women's Health Concern to continue to help women toward better health care.

Anyone needing information or practical help can write (sending SAE) to Women's Health Concern, at the above address.

The National Osteoporosis Society (NOS)
PO Box 10, Barton Meade House, Radstock, Bath, Avon (0761 32472)

Set up in 1986, this is a registered charity whose highly effective work is currently being backed to the tune of £80,000 by the DHSS. The current Chairman, Dr Allan Dixon, who has written the foreword to this book, helped to found NOS in 1986, in his own words 'to harness people power, to influence politicians and doctors regarding the magnitude of the national osteoporosis problem so that something would be done about it'. The Vice-Chairman is HRT pioneer, John Studd, consultant gynaecologist at King's College Hospital.

In three years, the society has grown to cover 10,000 members, all of them supporting the work and aims of the NOS. Some are already suffering from osteoporosis but others just want to learn how to reduce their risk of developing it. The number of 'professionals' among members, doctors, medical scientists, nurses and paramedics has become so great that a separate scientific branch of NOS has now been set up. Following an NOS initiative, the *International Journal of Osteo-*

porosis will shortly be launched and Britain is now joined to Europe in the European Foundation for Osteoporosis and Bone Disease.

Extremely readable and informative lay-level booklets and leaflets are available from NOS, and they can provide details of your nearest centre for osteoporosis treatment.

The annual modest membership fee of £5 a year (£3, if under eighteen) is nowhere near enough to cover administrative and postal costs, or for printing the booklets and regular newsletters sent to members. Funding is also needed for the vital work NOS does to help existing sufferers and to cover education on prevention among the public, the doctors and, above all, among children, which is where bone protection strategies should really begin. In addition to all this and to organizing local support groups, prime NOS aims include raising money for bone-scanning and research and for proper headquarters and training centre.

In a sense, NOS are victims of their own success and vision, and in November 1989, at the Royal Society of Medicine, they launched 'The Great British Bone Appeal' with a target of £1 million to fund and expand their work. The first donation received was from The Queen Mother.

The Amarant Trust

The Amarant Trust Membership Department, 16–24 Lonsdale Road, London NW6 6RD (081 200 0200)

Amarant was a mythical, never-fading flower, which was a symbol of immortality and enduring beauty to the Greeks. It was chosen as an appropriate name for a charitable trust set up in 1986, by Teresa Gorman MP and Malcolm Whitehead, consultant gynaecologist at King's College Hospital, who has been an outstanding pioneer of HRT in Britain. One of the aims of Amarant includes raising funds to enable the outstanding HRT and menopause research, carried out at King's College Hospital, to be continued and expanded.

In addition, however, Amarant aims to promote a better understanding of the menopause and the biological changes that occur in women from the mid-forties as hormone levels decline. At the same time, it sets out to alert women to the existence of HRT, which by replacing the missing hormones can combat these changes, restore the quality of life, eliminate menopause symptoms and, in particular, prevent the increased bone loss that can lead to post-menopausal osteoporosis.

At medical level this is done by a team of King's College specialists through post-graduate meetings and special study days for GPs (invariably over-subscribed). These offer the opportunity for the latest information on HRT techniques and research to be disseminated and for any prescribing or diagnostic problems to be discussed. This medical education work is now being extended to other health professionals.

At lay level, information and advice is available via leaflets, booklets, video and audio tapes as well as through ten special telephone helplines. Personal advice, assessment and treatment is also available at the Amarant Centre, a self- or GP-referral clinic manned by King's College doctors and sited at London's Churchill Clinic. Other additional services can also be obtained such as cervical smears, thyroid function tests, mammograms, etc. This is the first of many such self-referral centres planned as more resources become available.

A new and important facet of Amarant work, however, concerns the setting up of Amarant groups. These local support groups, now proliferating across the country, are designed to boost morale and increase understanding through exchange of information and experience. Anyone interested in joining such a group (or starting one in their own area) can apply to Amarant for information.

Although the work of the Amarant Trust is assisted by a modest DHSS grant, it relies for income mainly on membership fees and donations from private individuals and companies, plus money made on the sale of Amarant tapes, books and telephone helplines. Booklets and regular newsletters are mailed free to members, who can also take advantage of a telephone advice line manned by a specialist menopause counsellor. Full details can be obtained from The Amarant Trust Membership Department, at the above address.

Disabled Living Foundation
380–384 Harrow Road, London W9 2HU (071-289 6111)

This is a national information and resource centre, covering all the latest equipment for disabled people, with professional advisors on hand.

There are thirty similar centres across the country and an up-to-date list of these can be obtained from the Disabled Living Centre Council, at the above address.

List of menopause and HRT clinics

§   National Health Service (NHS)
#   Private
*   Charge made (on a non-profitmaking basis)

Aberdeen: § Dr Anderson, Aberdeen Royal Infirmary Foresthill, Aberdeen AB9 QZB (0224 681818)

Airdrie: § Mrs A White, Health Department, Adam Avenue, Airdrie (0236 69229)

Ashford: § Dr Stewart, Menopause Clinic, William Harvey Hospital, Kennington Road, Ashford, Kent (0233 633331)

Barnsley: § Dr Wunna, Menopause Advisory Clinic, Family Planning Clinic, Queens Road, Barnsley, South Yorkshire (0226 730000)

Barrow-in-Furness: § Dr Jill Tattersall, Well Woman Clinic, Atinson Road, Barrow-in-Furness, Cumbria (0229 27212)

Basingstoke: § Mrs Hemington, Fairfield's Clinic, Fairfield's Road, Basingstoke RG24 (0256 26980)

Beckenham: § Mr J McQueen, Gynaecology Department, Beckenham Hospital, 379 Croydon Road, Beckenham, Kent (081 650 0125)

Belfast: § Mr J. Houston, Samaritan Hospital, Lisburn Road, Belfast (0232 332300)

Birmingham: # Miss D. Gray, St Mary's Road, Harborne B17 0HA (021 427 6525)

    also: § Dr Gillian Stuart, Menopause Clinic, Maternity Hospital, Queen Elizabeth Medical Centre, Birmingham B15 2TG (021 472 1377)

    also: § Dr Gillian Stuart, Birmingham and Midland Hospital for Women, Showall Green Lane, Sparkhill, Birmingham B11 (021 722 1101)

178 Understanding Osteoporosis

also: # Dr Gillian Stuart, AMI Priory Hospital, 22 Priory Road, Edgbaston, Birmingham B5 7UG (021 440 6611)

also: # Dr Gillian Stuart, The Edgbaston Nuffield Hospital, 22 Somerset Road, Edgbaston, Birmingham B15 2QD (021 456 2000)

also: # Mr J. Jordan, 20 Church Road, Edgbaston, Birmingham B15 (021 454 2345)

also: § Dr P. Plant, Menopause Clinic, 5 York Road, Birmingham B16 9HH, (021 454 8236)

also: § Dr P. Plant, Menopause Counselling, St Patrick's Family Planning Clinic, Highgate Street, Birmingham B12 0YA (021 440 2422)

also: § Dr Mushin, Soho Health Centre, Louise Road, Handsworth, Birmingham (021 523 9231)

also: § Dr Threlfall, Warren Farm Health Centre, Warren Farm Road, Kingstanding, Birmingham (021 373 1740)

also: § Dr Threlfall and Dr Ahamed, Aston Health Centre, Trinity Road, Aston, Birmingham (021 328 7900)

also: § Dr Thake, Annie Wood Resource Centre, Alma Way, Lozells, Birmingham (021 554 7137/3155)

Bournemouth: # Dr Susan Parker, 2 Clarendon Road, Westbourne, Dorset BH4 8AH (0202 764803)

Brighton: § Mr Beard, Family Planning Clinic, Morely Street, Brighton, East Sussex BN2 2RA (0273 693600)

also: § Mr Malville, Royal Sussex Hospital, Eastern Road, Brighton, Sussex BN2 5BE (0273 696955)

Braintree: § St Michael's Day Hospital, Rayne Road, Braintree (0245 261749)

Bristol: # Dr Ruth Coles, Richmond Hill Clinic, 25 Denmark Street, Bristol BS1 5DQ (0272 292183)

Buckingham: § Dr Brown, Family Planning Clinic, Buckingham Hospital, Buckingham Town, Bucks MK18 1NU (0280 813243)

Burton-on-Trent: § Dr Naomi Spencer, Burton District Hospital, Belvedere Road, Burton-on-Trent, Staffordshire DE13 0RB (0283 66333)

also: § Dr Naomi Spencer, Bridge Street Surgery, 23 Bridge Street, Burton-on-Trent (0283 63451)

Chelmsford: § The Health Clinic, Springfield Green, Essex (0245 261749)

Chester: § Mr John Williams, Family Planning Clinic, Maternity Unit, Countess of Chester Hospital, Liverpool Road, Chester (0244 365000)

Consett: § Mr Johnson, Menopause Clinic, Out-patients Department, Shotley Bridge General Hospital, Shotley Bridge, Consett, Co Durham BH8 0NB (0207 503456)

Doncaster: § Health Centre, Crooksbroom Lane, Hatfield, Doncaster CN7 6JQ (0302 841373)

Dublin: * Rita Burtenshaw, Dublin Well Woman Centre, 73 Lower Lesson Street, Dublin 2 (610083/610086)

also: § Dr N. Cleary, Coombe Hospital, Dublin (537561)

also: # Ms H. Walsh, 59 Synge Street, Dublin 8 (780712)

also: # Dr Kearns, 5–7 Catbal Brugha Street, Dublin 1 (727726/723363)

Durham: § Dr Steel, Dryburn Hospital, North Road, Durham DH1 5TW (091 386 4911)

Edinburgh: § Dr J. Bancroft, Dean Terrace Centre, 18 Dean Terrace, Edinburgh EH4 1NL (031 332 7941/031 343 6243)

also: § Mr White, Edinburgh Royal Infirmary, 39 Chalmers Street, Edinburgh (031 229 2477)

Gateshead: Mr Silverstone, Queen Elizabeth Hospital, Gateshead, Tyne and Wear (091 487 8989)

Glasgow: § Dr Helen McEwan, Glasgow Royal Infirmary, Castle Street, Glasgow G4 0SF (041 552 3535)

also: § Dr David McKay Hart, Bone Metabolism Research Unit, Western Infirmary, Glasgow G11 6NT (041 339 8822)

also: § Dr David McKay Hart, Stobhill Hospital, Balornock Road, Glasgow G21 (041 558 0111)

also: § Dr E. Wilson, Family Planning Centre, 2 Claremont Terrace, Glasgow G3 (041 332 9411)

also: § Miss Fraser (Mondays 7.30 to 9.00p.m.), Central Health Centre, North Carbrain Road, Cumbernauld, Glasgow G67 1BJ (0236 731771)

Grimsby: § Winn Davey, Well Woman Centre, Eleanor Street, Grimsby, South Humberside (0472 362098)

Hatfield: # Dr Brenda Bean, Medical Centre, Hatfield Polytechnic College, College Lane, Hatfield, Herts (0707 279444)

Havant: # Dr Sarah Randall, BUPA Hospital, Portsmouth, Bartons Road, Havant, Hants PO9 5NP (0705 454511) *also*: § Dr Thomas, Menopausal Clinic, Havant Health Centre, Civic Centre Road, Havant PO9 2AZ (0705 455111)

High Wycombe: * Dr Chapman, The Wycombe Clinic, 6 Harlow Road, High Wycombe, Bucks HP13 6AA (0494 26666)

Hove: # Dr Jones, 32 Westbourne Villas, Hove, Sussex (0273 720217)

also: § Well Woman Clinic, Mortimer House, 12A Western Road, Hove, East Sussex (0273 774075)

Keighley: § Dr D. Miles, Airedale General Hospital, Steeton, Keighley, West Yorkshire BD20 6TD (0535 52511 x 442)

Kendal: § Dr Daphne Lowe, Well Woman Clinic, Blackhall Road, Kendal, Cumbria (0935 727564)

Kenilworth: § Dr Felicity Smith, Menopause Advice Clinic, Kenilworth Clinic, Smalley Place, Kenilworth, Warwickshire (0926 52087)

Leeds: § Dr Mary Jones, Clarendon Wing, Leeds General Infirmary, Belmont Grove, Leeds LS2 9NS (0532 432799 x 3886)

Liverpool: § Mrs Francis, Menopause Clinic, The Womens' Hospital, Catherine Street, Liverpool L8 7NJ (051 709 1000)

also: # Mr R. G. Farquharson, 31 Rodney Street, Liverpool L1 9EH (051 709 8522)

also: § Dr Carter, Cytology Department, Community Headquarters, Sefton General Hospital, Smithdown Road, Liverpool L15 2HE (051 733 4020 x 2555)

also: # Mr H. Francis, 25 Britannia Pavilion, Albert Dock, Liverpool L3 (051 709 3998)

London: § Mrs T. R. Varma, Consultant Gynaecologist, St George's Medical School and Hospital, Blackshaw Road, London SW17 (081 672 1255)

also: * Dr Kouba, Marie Stopes Clinic, 108 Whitfield Street, London W1 (071 388 0662/2585)

also: Dr Mary Griffin, PMT and Menopause Clinic, The London Hospital, Whitechapel, London E1 1BB (071 377 7000 x 2030)

also: § Dr Shamougan, Park Lane Clinic, 131 Park Lane, London N17 (081 808 9094) *also*: § Dr Nicholls, Crouch End Health Centre, 45 Middle Lane, London N8 (081 341 2045)

also: § Dr Shamougan, Stuart Crescent Health Centre, 8 Stuart Crescent, London N22 (081 889 4311)

also: # Mr N. Cullen, BUPA Screen Unit for Women, BUPA Medical Centre, Battle Bridge House, 300 Grays Inn Road, London WC1X 8DU (071 837 6484 x 2304)

also: § Mr Ballard, Queen Mary's Hospital, Roehampton Lane, Roehampton, London SW15 5PN (081 789 6611)

also: § Patrick Doody Clinic, Pelham Road, London SW19 (081 685 9922)

also * The Amarant Centre, 80 Lambeth Road, London SE1 7PW (071 401 3855)

also: # Mr John Studd, 120 Harley Street, London W1N 1AG (071 486 0497/7641)

also: # Mr John Studd, Lister Hospital, Chelsea Bridge Road, London SW1 (071 730 5433/3417)

also: § Mr John Studd, Dulwich Hospital, East Dulwich Grove, London SE5 (071 693 9236/3377)

also: § Mr Malcolm Whitehead, Menopause Clinic, Queen Charlottes Hospital, Goldhawk Road, London W6 0XG (081 740 3910)

also: § Mr Malcolm Whitehead, Menopause Clinic, King's College Hospital, Denmark Hill, London SE5 9RS (081 733 0224)

also: # Dr G. Chodhury, 886 Garratt Lane, London SW17 (081 648 3234)

also: § Mr P. Saunders, Menopause Clinic, Gynaecology Out-Patients Department, St Thomas Hospital, Lambeth Place Road, London SE1 (071 928 9292 x 2533)

also: # Dr C. Mortimer, Osteoporosis and Menopause Clinic, Endocrine and Dermatology Centre, 140 Harley Street, London W1N 1AH (071 935 2440)

also: § Mr Agarwal, Royal Free Hospital, Pond Street, London NW3 2QG (081 435 9693)

also: § Mrs M. Hickerton, Balham Health Centre, 120 Bedford Hill, London SW12 (081 673 1201, appointments, or 081 672 0317, advice)

also: § Professor Franks, Samaritan Hospital for Women, Marylebone Road, London NW1 5YE (071 402 4211) *also*: § Dr Boutwood, The Bloosmbury Menopause Clinic, Elizabeth Garrett Anderson Hospital for Women, 144 Euston Road, London NW1 (071 387 2501)

also: # Dr Hubinont, 9A Wilbraham Place, Sloane Street, London SW1X 9AL (071 730 7928)

also: # Dr Cram, 121 Harley Street, London W1 (071 935 7111)

also: # Miss Cardozo, 129 Harley Street, London W1 (071 935 2357)

also: # Dr Dean, 12 Thurloe Street, London SW7 (071 584 6204)

Macclesfield: § Dr Leslie Batchelor, Well Woman Clinic, Family Planning and Ante-natal Clinic, West Park Hospital, Macclesfield, Cheshire (0625 661169)

Maldon: § The Health Clinic, Wantz Chase, Maldon, Essex (0245 261749)

Manchester: § Mrs Gallimore, Ann Street Health Centre, Ann Street, Denton, Manchester M34 2AS (061 320 7000)

also: § Mr Dawe, North Manchester General Hospital, Delauney's Road, Crumpsall, Manchester M8 6RB (061 795 4567)

also: § Mrs B. Stevenson, Palatine Centre, 63–65 Palatine Road, Manchester M20 9LJ (061 434 3555)

also: § Dr Ann Webb, Wythenshaw Health Care Centre, Stancliff Road, Manchester M22 (061 437 4625)

Mexborough: § Mr Fenton, Mexborough Montagu Hospital, Adwick Road, Mexborough, South Yorkshire (0709 585171)

Moulsham Lodge: § The Health Clinic, Lilac Way, Gloucester Avenue, Moulsham Lodge, Essex (0245 261749)

New Barnet: § Dr Kay, Menopausal and Well Woman Clinic, East Barnet Health Centre, 149 East Barnet Road, New Barnet, Herts EN4 8QZ (081 440 1251)

Newcastle under Lyme: § Dr O'Brien, 14 Harrowby Drive, Newcastle under Lyme, Staffordshire (0782 614265)

Newcastle upon Tyne: § Dr Roger Francis, Department of Medicine, Newcastle General Hospital, Westgate Road, Newcastle upon Tyne NE4 6BE (091 273 8811)

North Cheam: § Priory Crescent Clinic, Priory Crescent, North Cheam, Surrey (081 685 9922)

Nottingham: § Dr Filshie, City Hospital, Hucknall Road, Nottingham (0602 691169)

Nuneaton: § Mr M. L. Cox, Gynaecology Out-Patient Department, George Elliot Hospital, College Street, Nuneaton CV10 7DJ (0203 384201 x 22675)

Oldham: § Mr A. M. Mander, The Royal Oldham Hospital, Rochdale Road, Oldham, Lancs OL1 2JH (061 624 0420)
also: # Mr A. M. Mander, Lancaster House, 174 Chamber Road, Oldham, Lancs OL8 4BY (061 652 1227)

Oxford: § Mr D. Barlow, The John Radcliffe Hospital, Headington, Oxford (0865 64711)

Peterborough: § Mr Hackman, Peterborough and District Hospital, Thorpe Road, Peterborough (0733 67451)

Plymouth: § Dr Falconer, Plymouth General Hospital, Freedom Field, Kensington Road, Plymouth PL4 7JJ (0752 668080)

Pontypool: § Dr A. Parker, Gwent Health Authority, Community Health Units, Block B, Caerleon House, Mantilard Park Estate, Pontypool, Gwent NP4 0AX (04955 57911)

Pontypridd: § Dr D. Pugh, East Glamorgan General Hospital, Church Village, Pontypridd, Mid-Glamorgan (0443 204242)

Portsmouth: § Dr Sarah Randall, The Ella Gordon Centre, East Wing, St Mary's Hospital, Portsmouth, Hampshire (0709 548680)

Rochdale: # Mr A. M. Mander, Highfield Private Hospital Place, Manchester Road, Rochdale, Lancs OL11 4LX (0706 55121)

Rotherham: # Mr K. J. Anderton, The Mews, Morthen Hall Lane, Morthen, Rotherham S66 6JL (0709 548680)

Rugby: § Mr A. D. Parsons, Menopausal Clinic, Hospital of St Cross, Barby Road, Rugby (0788 572831)

Scunthorpe: # Mr Heywood, The Crosby Nursing Home, 207 Fordingham Road, Scunthorpe, South Humberside (0724 721191)
also: § Miss Stringer, The Scunthorpe General Hospital, Cliff Gardens, Scunthorpe, South Yorkshire (0724 282282)

Sheffield: § Dr J. Wordsworth, Central Health Clinic, Mulberry Street, Sheffield S1 2PJ (0742 768885) *also*: § Dr Taylor, North General Hospital, Herries Road, Sheffield (0742 434343)

   also: § Miss B. Jackson, Family Planning Association, 17 North Church Street, Sheffield S1 (0742 721191)

   also: § Dr Wordsworth, Royal Hallamshire Hospital, Glossop Road, Sheffield (0742 766222)

Slough: § Dr June Lawson, Menopause Clinic, Slough Family Planning Clinic, Osborne Street, Slouth (0753 26875)

Solihull: § Mr D. Sturdee, Menopause Clinic, Department of Obstetrics and Gynaecology, Lode Lane, Solihull B91 2JL (021 711 4455)

South Woodham Ferrers: § The Health Clinic, Merchant Street, South Woodham Ferrers, Essex (0245 261749)

Stafford: § Mr A. B. Duke, HRT Clinic, Stafford District General Hospital, Western Road, Stafford (0785 57731)

Staines: § Mr P. Saunders, Ashford Hospital, Staines, Middlesex (0784 251188)

Stalybridge: § Mrs Brierley, Stalybridge Clinic, Stamford Street, Stalybridge, Cheshire (061 338 2728)

Stockport: § Stepping Hill Hospital, Stockport, Cheshire (061 483 1010)

Stockton-on-Tees: § Mrs W. Francis, Women's Health Advice Centre, 31 Yarm Lane, Stockton-on-Tees, Cleveland (0642 674393)

Stourbridge: § Mrs Widdett (counselling only), Wordsley Green Health Centre, Lawnsford Road, Wordsley, Stourbridge, West Midlands (0384 271271)

Sunderland: § Mrs Batts, Well Woman Clinic, Pallian Health Centre, Hylton Road, Sunderland (091 514 4166)

Sutton Coldfield: § Menopausal Counselling Clinic, Good Hope Hospital, Rectory Road, Sutton Coldfield, West Midlands, B75 7RR (021 378 2211)

Swansea: § Dr Anand, Central Clinic (counselling only), Trinity Building, 21 Orchard Street, Swansea (0792 651791)

   also: § Mr P. Bowen-Simpkins (monthly), Gynaecology Department, Singleton Hospital, Sketty, Swansea SA2 8QA (0792 205666)

Tunbridge Wells: § Family Planning Clinic, 21 Dudley Road, Tunbridge Wells, Kent TN1 1LE (0892 30002)

Uxbridge: § Dr Walefield (counselling only), Uxbridge Health Centre, George Street, Uxbridge, Middlesex (0895 52461)

Ware: # Mrs Rita Harrison, Health Centre, Bowling Road, Ware, Herts (0920 50705)

Warrington: # Dr Marjorie Monks, Private Care, (Counselling and Women's) 29 Wilson Pattern Street, Warrington WA1 1PG (0925 50705)

Wednesbury: § Alison Day, Mesty Croft Clinic, Alma Street, Wednesbury, West Midlands (021 556 0020)

Wendover: § Pat Hancock, Wendover Health Centre, Aylesbury Road, Wendover, Bucks (0296 623452)

Wimborne: § Dr De Silva (Counselling only), Wimborne Clinic, Rowlands Hill, Wimborne, Dorset BH21 1AR (0202 882405)

Worcester: § Dr Joan Windsor, St John's Clinic, Family and Preventative Care Services Unit, 1 Bromyard Road, Worcester WR2 5BS (0905 424979)

Many hospitals which do not run special menopause clinics, and are not, therefore, listed here, will accept menopause and osteoporosis referrals within their obstetric and gynaecology departments. In most large hospitals, at least one gynaecologist or endocrinologist has a special interest in HRT. A referral letter is required in all cases under NHS and *preferred* for private consultations with a gynaecologist or at private clinics. If you are seen without GP referral, your doctor will be informed retrospectively. The names of the doctors running the listed clinics may change from time to time, but those given were correct in March 1990.

Anyone encountering difficulties in obtaining treatment should contact The Amarant Trust, Women's Health Concern or the National Osteoporosis Society. FPA Headquarters, at 27–35 Mortimer Street, London, W1N 7RJ (071 636 7866), will also advise, and can give the name of the nearest menopause clinic for any area in the country.

Remember you have the right to ask for a second opinion, or the right to change your doctor, if this should prove necessary. You should expect to share in discussion and decisions concerning your health, your body and your bones.

Further reading

The menopause and HRT
No Change, (7th edition) by Wendy Cooper (Arrow, 1990)
The Amarant Book of HRT, by Teresa Gorman and Dr Malcolm Whitehead (Pan, 1989)
The Menopause, (A Women's Health Concern Publication, 1985)
What Every Woman Needs to Know about Osteoporosis and Hormone Replacement Therapy (An NOS publication, 1989)

Cystitis
Understanding Cystitis, by Angela Kilmartin (Arrow, 1986)
Sexual Cystitis, by Angela Kilmartin (Arrow, 1988)

Nutrition
The Calcium Guide Book (An NOS publication; free to members, £2 to non-members; published anually)
The Dictionary of Nutritional Health, by Adrienne Mayes PhD (Thorsons, 1986)
The Food Factor, (6th edition) by Barbara Griggs (Penguin, 1988)

The Contraceptive Pill
Everything You Need to Know about the Pill, by Wendy Cooper and Dr Tom Smith (Sheldon, 1984)

Hysterectomy
Hysterectomy, by Suzie Hayman (Sheldon, 1986)

Your Heart
Heart and Cardio-vascular Protection
Living with High Blood Pressure, by Dr Tom Smith (Sheldon, 1985)
? with your Heart, by Dr Tom Smith (Sheldon, 1990)

Index